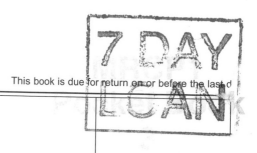

Clinical Pharmacology
Endocrinology
Gastroenterology
Nephrology

Third Edition

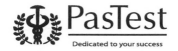

PasTest

Dedicated to your success

MRCP1
Pocket Book
3

Clinical Pharmacology
Endocrinology
Gastroenterology
Nephrology

Simon Constable BSc MB BS MRCP(UK) PGCert (LTHE)
Colin M Dayan MA FRCP PhD
Peter Collins MD MRCP
Helen Paynter MBChB DRCOG MRCP MA

Third Edition

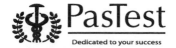

PasTest
Dedicated to your success

© 2008 PASTEST LTD
Egerton Court, Parkgate Estate
Knutsford, Cheshire, WA16 8DX
Telephone: 01565 752000

Third edition 2008
Second edtion 2004
First edition 2002
Reprinted 2009

ISBN: 1 905635 05 2
ISBN: 978 1 905635 05 4

A catalogue record for this book is available from the British Library.

The information contained within this book was obtained by the author from reliable sources. However, while every effort has been made to ensure its accuracy, no responsibility for loss, damage or injury occasioned to any person acting or refraining from action as a result of information contained herein can be accepted by the publishers or author.

PasTest Revision Books and Intensive Courses

PasTest has been established in the field of postgraduate medical education since 1972, providing revision books and intensive study courses for doctors preparing for their professional examinations.

Books and courses are available for the following specialties:
MRCGP, MRCP Parts 1 and 2, MRCPCH Parts 1 and 2, MRCS, MRCOG Parts 1 and 2, DRCOG, DCH, FRCA, Dentistry.

For further details contact:
PasTest, Freepost, Knutsford, Cheshire WA16 7BR
Tel: 01565 752000   Fax: 01565 650264
www.pastest.co.uk   enquiries@pastest.co.uk

Text prepared by Keytec Typesetting Ltd, Bridport, Dorset
Printed and bound in the UK by CPI Antony Rowe

CONTENTS

INTRODUCTION

PasTest's MRCP Part 1 Pocket Books are designed to help the busy examination candidate to make the most of every opportunity to revise. With this little book in your pocket, it is the work of a moment to open it, choose a question, decide upon your answers and then check the answer. Revising 'on the run' in this manner is both reassuring (if your answer is correct) and stimulating (if you find any gaps in your knowledge).

The MRCP Part 1 examination consists of two papers, each lasting three hours. Both papers contain 100 'Best of Five' questions (one answer is chosen from five options). Questions in each specialty are randomised across both papers. *No marks are deducted for a wrong answer.*

One-best-answer/'Best of Five' MCQs
An important characteristic of one-best-answer MCQs is that they can be designed to test application of knowledge and clinical problem-solving rather than just the recall of facts. This should change (for the better) the ways in which candidates prepare for MRCP Part 1.

Each one-best MCQ has a question stem, which usually contains clinical information, followed by five branches. All five branches are typically homologous (eg all diagnoses, all laboratory investigations, all antibiotics etc) and should be set out in a logical order (eg alphabetical). Candidates are asked to select the ONE branch that is the best answer to the question. A response is not required to the other four branches. The answer sheet is, therefore, slightly different from that used for true/false MCQs.

A good strategy that can be used with many well-written one-best MCQs is to try to reach the correct answer without first scrutinising the five options. If you can then find the answer you have reached in the option list, then you are probably correct.

One-best-answer MCQs are quicker to answer than multiple true/false MCQs because only one response is needed for each question. Even though the question stem for onebest-answer MCQs is usually longer than for true/false questions, and therefore takes a little longer to read carefully, it is reasonable to set more one-best than true/false MCQs for the same exam duration – in this instance 60 true/false and 100 one-best are used in exams of 2 hours' duration.

Application of Knowledge and Clinical Problem-Solving
Unlike true/false MCQs, which test mainly the recall of knowledge, one-best-answer questions test application and problem-solving. This makes them more effective test items and is one of the reasons why testing time can be reduced. In

order to answer these questions correctly, it is necessary to apply basic knowledge – not just the ability to remember it. Furthermore, candidates who cannot reach the correct answer by applying their knowledge are much less likely to be able to choose the right answer by guessing than they were with true/false MCQs. This gives a big advantage to the best candidates, who have good knowledge and can apply it in clinical situations.

Books like the ones in this series, which consist of 'Best of Five' questions in subject categories, can help you to focus on specific topics and to isolate your weaknesses. You should plan a revision timetable to help you spread your time evenly over the range of subjects likely to appear in the examination. PasTest's **Essential Revision Notes for MRCP** by P Kalra will provide you with essential notes on all aspects of the syllabus.

CONTRIBUTORS

THIRD EDITION

Clinical Pharmacology
Simon Constable BSc MB BS MRCP(UK) PGCert (LTHE) Medical Director, Manchester Clinical Research Unit, ICON Development Solutions, Honorary Senior Lecturer in Clinical Pharmacology, The University of Liverpool Honorary Consultant Physician, Royal Liverpool and Broadgreen University Hospitals NHS Trust

Endocrinology
Colin M Dayan MA FRCP PhD, Consultant Senior Lecturer in Medicine, Head of Clinical Research, Henry Wellcome Laboratories for Integrative Neuroscience and Endocrinology, University of Bristol, Bristol.

Gastroenterology
Peter Collins MD MRCP, Consultant Hepatologist, Bristol Royal Infirmary, Bristol.

Nephrology
Helen Paynter MBChB DRCOG MRCP MA Associate Specialist in Nephrology, Princess of Wales Hospital, Bridgend.

SECOND EDITION

Clinical Pharmacology – Pocket Book 4
Professor M Pirmohamed PhD FRCP FRCP (Edin) Professor of Clinical Pharmacology and Hon Consultant Physician, Department of Pharmacology and Therapeutics, University of Liverpool, Liverpool.

Endocrinology
Colin M Dayan MA FRCP PhD, Consultant Senior Lecturer in Medicine, Head of Clinical Research, Henry Wellcome Laboratories for Integrative Neuroscience and Endocrinology, University of Bristol, Bristol.

Gastroenterology
Timothy Heymann MA MBA FRCP, Consultant Physician and Gastroenterology, Kingston Hospital, Surrey.
Christopher S J Probert MD FRCPILTM, University of Medicine, Bristol Royal Infirmary, Bristol.

Nephrology
Julian R Wright MB BS BSC(Hons) MRCP, Specialist Registrar, Department of Renal Medicine, Manchester Royal Infirmary, Manchester.
Helen Paynter MRCP, Staff Grade Renal & General Medicine, Gloucestershire Royal Hospital, Gloucester.

Clinical Pharmacology

Best of Five

Questions

CLINICAL PHARMACOLOGY: 'BEST OF FIVE' QUESTIONS

For each of the questions select the ONE most appropriate answer from the options provided.

1.1   A 70-year-old woman with type 2 diabetes mellitus is found to have impaired renal function on routine testing. She has recently been treated for a urinary tract infection. She is on a number of different medications (listed below). Which drug could potentially be a possible cause of her deterioration in renal function?

☐   **A**   Atenolol
☐   **B**   Diclofenac
☐   **C**   Digoxin
☐   **D**   Metformin
☐   **E**   Trimethoprim

1.2   A 43-year-old female patient has recently been diagnosed as having acute intermittent porphyria. She asks you for clarification about which drugs are safe for her to have in the future. Which of the following drugs are considered safe for use in such patients?

☐   **A**   Carbamazepine
☐   **B**   Co-amoxiclav
☐   **C**   Erythromycin
☐   **D**   Gliclazide
☐   **E**   Simvastatin

1.3   A 60-year-old woman with hypertension and trigeminal neuralgia sees her dentist because of gingival hypertrophy. The dentist considers whether one of her medications (listed below) is responsible. Which one of these drugs is the most likely culprit?

☐   **A**   Atenolol
☐   **B**   Bendroflumethiazide
☐   **C**   Carbamazepine
☐   **D**   Nifedipine
☐   **E**   Perindopril

1.4   A 70-year-old man is treated with warfarin for chronic atrial fibrillation. He also has chronic obstructive pulmonary disease and develops a community-acquired pneumonia, requiring antibiotic therapy. Which of the following antibiotics should be used with caution in this man because of a potential pharmacokinetic interaction with warfarin?

- ☐ **A** Amoxicillin
- ☐ **B** Ceftriaxone
- ☐ **C** Co-amoxiclav
- ☐ **D** Erythromycin
- ☐ **E** Trimethoprim

1.5   A 30-year-old HIV-positive man is being treated with antiretrovirals. A new drug is started and within the first 6 weeks he develops what is believed to be a hypersensitivity reaction characterized by a rash, fever and diarrhoea. Which of the following drugs must be considered as a potential causative agent and stopped immediately?

- ☐ **A** Abacavir
- ☐ **B** Didanosine
- ☐ **C** Efavirenz
- ☐ **D** Nevirapine
- ☐ **E** Saquinavir

1.6   A 75-year-old man with ischaemic heart disease is treated with amiodarone for paroxysmal non-sustained ventricular tachycardia. Which of the following statements about amiodarone therapy is true?

- ☐ **A** Steady-state plasma concentrations of amiodarone will be achieved within a week of the initiation of oral therapy
- ☐ **B** Amiodarone has a relatively small apparent volume of distribution
- ☐ **C** Amiodarone has β-adrenoceptor blocking activity
- ☐ **D** The development of corneal microdeposits is rare
- ☐ **E** Pulmonary fibrosis occurs only during long-term use of the drug

Answers on pages 83–102

1.7   A 62-year-old diabetic man with hypertension attends his GP
       complaining of gynaecomastia. Which of his following drugs is most
       likely to be responsible for this adverse effect?

    □ **A** Amlodipine
    □ **B** Enalapril
    □ **C** Furosemide
    □ **D** Gliclazide
    □ **E** Metformin

1.8   A 70-year-old woman is commenced on dalteparin during the
       investigation and subsequent initial treatment of a pulmonary embolus.
       Warfarin is added after 5 days but the patient takes several more days to
       achieve a therapeutic international normalised ratio (INR) and the
       dalteparin is eventually stopped after 10 days. Which particular adverse
       effect should medical staff have vigilance for in this patient?

    □ **A** Hepatitis
    □ **B** Hypokalaemia
    □ **C** Osteoporosis
    □ **D** Leucopoenia
    □ **E** Thrombocytopenia

1.9   A 65-year-old woman with a number of different medical problems
       becomes jaundiced and after extensive investigations the hepatologists
       conclude that this is drug related. Her liver function tests show a
       bilirubin of 80 µmol/l, alanine aminotransferase 46 IU, gamma-glutamyl
       transferase 385 IU and alkaline phosphatase 450 IU. Which of her
       following drugs is the most likely culprit under these circumstances?

    □ **A** Amiodarone
    □ **B** Chlorpromazine
    □ **C** Metformin
    □ **D** Omeprazole
    □ **E** Rosiglitazone

1.10 A consultant psychiatrist decides to use lithium in the treatment of a female patient with bipolar disorder. The doctor considers a number of factors before initiating the prescription and advising the patient and her GP. Which one of the following pieces of advice is most applicable?

- ☐ **A** Therapeutic drug monitoring is not required unless the patient is taking diuretic therapy
- ☐ **B** The dose of lithium should be adjusted to maintain serum lithium concentrations above 2 mmol/l
- ☐ **C** Renal and thyroid function should be monitored at least once a year
- ☐ **D** There are no long-term consequences for cognitive function for patients on chronic lithium therapy
- ☐ **E** Weight loss is a common problem

1.11 A 40-year-old woman attends a clinic for medical disorders in pregnancy. She has cardiovascular disease and is discussing the options for anticoagulation during her (unplanned) pregnancy and breast feeding. Which of the following drugs (at normal therapeutic doses) would be contraindicated in pregnancy because they may be harmful to the baby in a mother who is breast-feeding?

- ☐ **A** Aspirin
- ☐ **B** Clopidogrel
- ☐ **C** Dalteparin
- ☐ **D** Unfractionated heparin
- ☐ **E** Warfarin

1.12 A 13-year-old child has been diagnosed with Stevens–Johnson syndrome. Which one of the following drugs is the most likely culprit?

- ☐ **A** Carbamazepine
- ☐ **B** Codeine
- ☐ **C** Lidocaine
- ☐ **D** Loratadine
- ☐ **E** Thyroxine

Answers on pages 83–102

1.13   A 45-year-old lady is admitted to the accident and emergency department slightly confused, with dilated pupils and a broad complex tachycardia on the electrocardiogram (ECG). Which of the following is the most likely culprit drug taken in overdose?

☐   **A**   Amitriptyline

☐   **B**   Clozapine

☐   **C**   Fluoxetine

☐   **D**   Haloperidol

☐   **E**   Lithium

1.14   A ward pharmacist draws your attention to a set of drug prescription charts, worried about a potentially clinically significant drug interaction? Which one of the following combinations of drugs gives rise to most concern?

☐   **A**   Digoxin and atorvastatin

☐   **B**   Carbamazepine and clobazam

☐   **C**   Erythromycin and amoxicillin

☐   **D**   Ciprofloxacin and theophylline

☐   **E**   Tramadol and codeine

1.15   Pharmacovigilance in the United Kingdom is currently supervised by which of the following bodies?

☐   **A**   Committee on Safety of Medicines (CSM)

☐   **B**   Commission on Human Medicines (CHM)

☐   **C**   National Institute for Health and Clinical Excellence (NICE)

☐   **D**   National Patient Safety Agency (NPSA)

☐   **E**   Medicines Control Agency (MCA)

1.16 **A 28-year-old homosexual man with a diagnosis of HIV infection is started on protease inhibitor in combination with abacavir and lamivudine for treatment. The physician counsels him and warns him about the possible occurrence of lipodystrophy with protease inhibitors. Lipodystrophy caused by protease inhibitors is characterised by which one of the following?**

- ☐ **A** Hypoglycaemia
- ☐ **B** Insulin resistance
- ☐ **C** Uveitis
- ☐ **D** Peripheral neuropathy
- ☐ **E** Renal failure

1.17 **You are in charge of an antenatal clinic and are frequently consulted by midwives in relation to the possible teratogenic effects of drugs being taken by pregnant women. Which one of the following drugs has been proved to have teratogenic effects in pregnant women?**

- ☐ **A** Diazepam
- ☐ **B** Misoprostol
- ☐ **C** Heparin
- ☐ **D** Oral contraceptives
- ☐ **E** Aspirin

1.18 **A 50-year-old woman consults you about the possibility of starting hormone replacement therapy (HRT). You discuss the benefits and risks of HRT. Which one of the following statements regarding HRT is true?**

- ☐ **A** Unopposed oestrogens should not be used in patients who have had a hysterectomy
- ☐ **B** It is associated with a two-fold increased risk of breast cancer
- ☐ **C** Conventional forms of hormone replacement therapy are less effective than newer compounds such as raloxifene
- ☐ **D** Its use increases the risk of Alzheimer's disease
- ☐ **E** The benefits on bone are the same irrespective of when the drugs are started after the menopause

Answers on pages 83–102

1.19 A 27-year-old woman presents with an overdose of a number of drugs that she has taken from the bathroom cabinet at home. Which one of the following is the most important consideration in her management?

☐ **A** Gastric lavage should be used up to 6 hours after the overdose

☐ **B** Ipecacuanha syrup should be used routinely

☐ **C** Activated charcoal reduces the enterohepatic circulation of drugs

☐ **D** Haemodialysis is useful for eliminating drugs with a high volume of distribution

☐ **E** Alkalinisation of urine should be used in all patients who have taken an aspirin overdose

1.20 You are asked to see a 30-year-old woman with hypertension who has peculiar dietary habits. In particular, she drinks 2 litres of grapefruit juice per day. You are concerned that this may lead to a serious interaction with which one of the following drugs that she is taking?

☐ **A** Perindopril

☐ **B** Ciclosporin

☐ **C** Atenolol

☐ **D** Bendroflumethiazide

☐ **E** Sodium valproate

1.21 A 70-year-old man presents with depression that you feel needs drug treatment. You choose to use fluoxetine, but the product information reveals that it undergoes extensive drug metabolism. Which one of the following statements concerning the process of drug metabolism is correct?

☐ **A** The primary role of drug metabolism is to convert hydrophilic compounds into lipophilic compounds

☐ **B** Drugs are only metabolised in the liver

☐ **C** Metabolism leads to the inactivation of fluoxetine

☐ **D** Cytochrome P450 enzymes are largely responsible for the phase II metabolic pathways

☐ **E** Genetically determined deficiencies of some of the drug metabolising enzymes have been described

1.22 **A 20-year-old man presents with symptoms of schizophrenia. In deciding on which drug to use, you consider that atypical neuroleptics in comparison to typical neuroleptics are generally:**

☐ **A** Less likely to cause parkinsonism

☐ **B** More likely to cause neuroleptic malignant syndrome

☐ **C** Less likely to affect the negative symptoms of schizophrenia

☐ **D** Less likely to affect the positive symptoms of schizophrenia

☐ **E** Less likely to cause weight gain

1.23 **A 2-year-old child develops infantile spasms and is started on vigabatrin by the paediatric neurologist. The mode of action of vigabatrin is thought to be through which one of the following?**

☐ **A** Glutamate antagonism

☐ **B** Inhibition of gamma aminobutyric acid (GABA) re-uptake

☐ **C** Inhibition of calcium conductance

☐ **D** Inhibition of sodium conductance

☐ **E** Inhibition of GABA transaminase

1.24 **A 30-year-old man with bipolar depression is started on lithium carbonate. Which one of the following statements is correct for this drug?**

☐ **A** It affects mood in normal subjects

☐ **B** It can cause central diabetes insipidus

☐ **C** It interacts with bendroflumethiazide (bendrofluazide)

☐ **D** It can be used in breast-feeding mothers

☐ **E** It can be used without dose alteration in patients with moderate to severe renal impairment

1.25 **A 46-year-old man develops an acute attack of gout, which is treated with high-dose diclofenac. Which one of the following drugs may be used safely in this patient without any risk of precipitating gout?**

☐ **A** Allopurinol

☐ **B** Probenecid

☐ **C** Atenolol

☐ **D** Adenosine

☐ **E** Ciclosporin

Answers on pages 83–102

1.26   **On a typical infectious diseases ward round you see many patients with different infections and on a variety of antibiotics. Regarding the use of antibiotics, which one of the following is a known characteristic?**

☐   **A**   Clindamycin is not used in the treatment of osteomyelitis because it does not penetrate bone well

☐   **B**   Clindamycin can be used for the treatment of pseudomembranous colitis

☐   **C**   Co-amoxiclav is effective against methicillin-resistant *Staphylococcus aureus*

☐   **D**   Amoxicillin is well known to cause cholestatic hepatitis

☐   **E**   Clarithromycin is active against atypical mycobacteria

1.27   **A 75-year-old woman on digoxin presents to the Emergency Department with nausea, vomiting and palpitations, which you feel may be due to digoxin toxicity. Which one of the following statements regarding digoxin toxicity is true?**

☐   **A**   It is potentiated by hypocalcaemia

☐   **B**   It is potentiated by hyponatraemia

☐   **C**   It is diagnosed by ST elevation on an electrocardiogram (ECG)

☐   **D**   It is treated with phenytoin

☐   **E**   It is treated with an infusion of calcium chloride

1.28   **A 72-year-old man is diagnosed with motor neurone disease and is started on riluzole. Which one of the following is a known feature of riluzole?**

☐   **A**   It acts as a glutamate agonist

☐   **B**   It can only be used in amyotrophic lateral sclerosis

☐   **C**   It improves functional capacity in patients with amyotrophic lateral sclerosis

☐   **D**   It causes an increase in liver enzymes in more than 1 in 1000 patients

☐   **E**   It has been shown to improve quality of life

1.29 **On a routine ward round you come across a 30-year-old diabetic patient on several drugs which you think act via receptors. Which one of the following is correct regarding receptor action?**

- ☐ **A** Receptors are present only on the plasma membrane
- ☐ **B** Receptors initiate the pharmacological actions of all drugs
- ☐ **C** Receptor actions remain constant in the continued presence of an agonist
- ☐ **D** Receptors interacting with G proteins usually stimulate guanylate cyclase activity
- ☐ **E** Insulin receptors are linked to transmembrane protein tyrosine kinases

1.30 **A 45-year-old man presents with epigastric pain and is diagnosed as having a duodenal ulcer on endoscopy. Biopsy of the duodenum shows the presence of *Helicobacter pylori*. Which one of the following statements is true regarding infection of the stomach by *H. pylori*?**

- ☐ **A** There is no need to eradicate *H. pylori* in patients with peptic ulcer
- ☐ **B** Patients with non-specific dyspepsia have been shown to benefit from eradication therapy
- ☐ **C** Long-term therapy with omeprazole without antibiotics can alter the distribution of infection within the stomach
- ☐ **D** The different eradication therapies are generally associated with an eradication rate of 70%
- ☐ **E** It is associated with an increase risk of cancer of the duodenum

1.31 **A 27-year-old with a long history of intravenous drug use presents with increased transaminases. He is diagnosed as being hepatitis C positive and the hepatologist decides to use interferon-α and ribavirin for treatment. Which one of the following is true regarding the use of interferon-α in chronic hepatitis C virus (HCV) infection?**

- ☐ **A** A sustained response rate is seen in 50% of patients
- ☐ **B** Fever is a rare adverse effect
- ☐ **C** It can lead to bone marrow suppression
- ☐ **D** Response is better in patients who are currently abusing alcohol
- ☐ **E** The concomitant use of paracetamol is contraindicated

Answers on pages 83–102

1.32 A 27-year-old woman presents to the Emergency Department after taking 48 Anadin® tablets. Which one of the following symptoms would you expect to find in this patient?

☐ **A** Tinnitus

☐ **B** Hyperglycaemia

☐ **C** Metabolic alkalosis

☐ **D** Peptic ulceration

☐ **E** Hypercoagulability

1.33 A 20-year-old schizophrenic patient is started on chlorpromazine. He presents 4 weeks later feeling unwell and is diagnosed as having neuroleptic malignant syndrome. Which one of the following statements is true regarding neuroleptic malignant syndrome?

☐ **A** It is a dose-related adverse effect of phenothiazines

☐ **B** Affected patients are fully conscious

☐ **C** Calcium-channel blockers have been shown to reduce mortality

☐ **D** It is characterised by elevated troponin T levels

☐ **E** It has an insidious onset

1.34 A 68-year-old man presents with acute atrial fibrillation. Which one of the following is true regarding the treatment of atrial fibrillation?

☐ **A** Adenosine is beneficial in the treatment of atrial fibrillation

☐ **B** Digoxin should be the first-line therapy in paroxysmal atrial fibrillation

☐ **C** Sotalol has class II (β-blocking) effects only

☐ **D** Propafenone has β-adrenoceptor-blocking activity

☐ **E** Magnesium may be of use in patients with rapid atrial fibrillation

1.35 You are asked to perform an audit on drug–drug interactions. On reviewing your notes you come up with the following combinations that were prescribed in patients. Which one of the following combinations would you consider to be harmful?

☐ **A** Rifabutin and clarithromycin

☐ **B** Zidovudine and aciclovir

☐ **C** Isosorbide mononitrate and atenolol

☐ **D** Aspirin and streptokinase

☐ **E** Naproxen and penicillamine

1.36 A 26-year-old epileptic patient on carbamazepine develops toxic epidermal necrolysis which necessitates intensive treatment in the intensive care unit (ITU) and a 6-week hospital stay. You decide to report this reaction on a yellow adverse drug reaction (ADR) reporting form. Which one of the following statements regarding ADR reporting in the UK is correct?

☐ **A** ADR reporting is compulsory

☐ **B** All serious ADRs should be reported

☐ **C** A black triangle (▼) sign by a drug in the *British National Formulary* (BNF) indicates that only allergic reactions need be reported

☐ **D** Only doctors, dentists and coroners are allowed to report on yellow cards

☐ **E** Yellow card reports allow a causal relationship to be established between a drug and an ADR

1.37 A 30-year-old man who weighs 70 kg presents with a large aspirin overdose. Haemodialysis is a treatment modality, the success of which will depend on the apparent volume of distribution (Vd). Which one of the following statements about Vd is correct in this man?

☐ **A** Vd does not exceed the volume of total body water

☐ **B** Vd would be expected to be 25 litres if the drug remained in the blood

☐ **C** Overdose of a drug with a high Vd can be treated by haemodialysis

☐ **D** Vd is low if the drug is avidly bound in the tissues

☐ **E** Vd can be calculated from a knowledge of the dose and concentration in plasma if the drug demonstrates linear kinetics

1.38   **A 20-year-old lady presents with weight loss, tremor, sweating and goitre. A clinical diagnosis of thyrotoxicosis is made and is confirmed by a suppressed thyroid stimulating hormone (TSH) level. Which one of the following is true regarding the use of antithyroid drugs?**

☐ **A**   Carbimazole inhibits the peripheral conversion of T_4 to T_3

☐ **B**   β-Blockers reduce the basal metabolic rate

☐ **C**   Carbimazole produces an improvement in 2 days

☐ **D**   Iodide can cause a goitre in euthyroid patients

☐ **E**   Radioactive iodine (^{131}I) predominantly emits gamma rays

1.39   **A 26-year-old man presents with methanol poisoning. Which one of the following is a known feature of poisoning with methanol?**

☐ **A**   The major route of elimination of methanol is via the kidneys

☐ **B**   Optic atrophy occurs within a few days

☐ **C**   Monitoring of blood levels is not required

☐ **D**   Metabolic acidosis with a normal anion gap is the usual finding

☐ **E**   Ethanol prevents methanol toxicity by inhibiting its oxidation within the liver

1.40   **A 40-year-old alcoholic man presents to your clinic complaining of the recent onset of flushing when alcohol is consumed. Which one of the following drugs is most likely to be responsible for this adverse effect?**

☐ **A**   Propranolol

☐ **B**   Chlorpromazine

☐ **C**   Thiamine

☐ **D**   Metronidazole

☐ **E**   Naltrexone

1.41 **Your hospital is drawing up new guidelines for the management of patients admitted with venous thromboembolism. One area for consideration is the use of low-molecular-weight heparins instead of unfractionated heparin. Low-molecular-weight heparins in comparison to unfractionated heparin are:**

☐ **A** Weaker inhibitors of thrombin

☐ **B** Less likely to have reduced clearance in patients with renal failure

☐ **C** Less likely to cause bleeding

☐ **D** More likely to cause thrombocytopenia

☐ **E** More likely to cause osteoporosis during long-term administration

1.42 **A 70-year-old woman presents with breast cancer. After surgery the patient is started on an aromatase inhibitor. Which one of the following is true regarding the use of aromatase inhibitors?**

☐ **A** Anastrozole is a less potent inhibitor than aminoglutethimide

☐ **B** Corticosteroid replacement is necessary in patients on aminoglutethimide

☐ **C** Anastrozole affects adrenal function

☐ **D** They are efficacious in premenopausal and postmenopausal women

☐ **E** Inhibition of aromatase occurs predominantly within the ovaries rather than in extraglandular sites

1.43 **A 45-year-old man with a body mass index of 33 kg/m^2 has failed to lose weight on various diet and exercise programmes and is considered for antiobesity drug therapy. Which one of the following statements regarding obesity and its treatment is correct?**

☐ **A** Sibutramine can be used in patients with hypertension

☐ **B** Heart valve regurgitation has been shown to be associated with treatment with fenfluramine and phentermine

☐ **C** Mitral stenosis occurs in association with the use of fenfluramine and phentermine

☐ **D** Selective serotonin re-uptake inhibitors cause heart valve abnormalities

☐ **E** Obesity *per se* is associated with a high prevalence of heart valve regurgitation

Answers on pages 83–102

1.44 A 46-year-old man presents to the Emergency Department with a painful erection, which is diagnosed as priapism. The attending physician feels that it is due to a drug that was started 3 weeks previously. Which one of the following drugs is associated with priapism?

□ **A** Trazodone

□ **B** Imipramine

□ **C** Captopril

□ **D** Atenolol

□ **E** Digoxin

1.45 A 6-year-old boy presents with an unintentional overdose of iron tablets. He is treated with antidotal therapy. Which one of the following is known to be an antidote for iron?

□ **A** Vitamin C

□ **B** Activated charcoal

□ **C** Desferrioxamine

□ **D** Fomepizole

□ **E** Dicobalt edetate

1.46 Which one of the following actions is mediated by the α-adrenoceptor?

□ **A** Bronchiolar constriction

□ **B** Decrease in gut motility

□ **C** Dilation of the splanchnic circulation

□ **D** Penile erection

□ **E** Relaxation of the pregnant uterus

1.47 Zanamivir in the treatment of influenza is characterised by all of the following, except:

□ **A** A bioavailability of less than 20%

□ **B** A decrease in bronchial air flow

□ **C** Increased release of virus from cells

□ **D** Reduced penetration of the virus into the respiratory mucosa

□ **E** Reduced severity of the illness

1.48   Cephalosporins:

☐ **A** Can be used in the treatment of *Clostridium difficile* diarrhoea

☐ **B** Can cause neutropenia and thrombocytopenia

☐ **C** Do not have a β-lactam ring in their structure

☐ **D** Have a 90% chance of causing allergy if the patient has had a previous reaction to penicillin

☐ **E** In general have half-lives greater than ten hours

1.49   Which one of the following causes of hypercalcaemia is most likely to respond to treatment with corticosteroids?

☐ **A** Milk-alkali syndrome

☐ **B** Paget's disease

☐ **C** Primary hyperparathyroidism

☐ **D** Sarcoidosis

☐ **E** Small-cell lung cancer

1.50   In relation to morphine, which one of the following statements is true?

☐ **A** Approximately 8% of the population cannot convert codeine to morphine

☐ **B** Morphine is more water soluble than diamorphine

☐ **C** Normal-release morphine has an onset of action within 5 minutes

☐ **D** Peak drug levels after once-daily preparations of morphine are reached after 12 hours

☐ **E** Pupillary constriction is an effect that is subject to tolerance

1.51   Regarding β-adrenoceptor antagonists:

☐ **A** Atenolol is a cardiospecific drug

☐ **B** Celiprolol increases total peripheral resistance

☐ **C** Drugs with intrinsic sympathomimetic activity are less likely to cause bradycardia

☐ **D** Esmolol is a long-acting drug used to treat patients with atrial arrhythmias

☐ **E** Propranolol causes prolongation of the QT interval

Answers on pages 83–102

1.52   **Which one of the following is a known effect of the anticonvulsant phenytoin?**

☐ **A**   Can cause selective IgA deficiency

☐ **B**   Causes arrhythmias in 10% of patients

☐ **C**   Displays first-order kinetics

☐ **D**   Efficacy in myoclonic epilepsy

☐ **E**   Osteoporosis is a known adverse effect

1.53   **The following are well-known drug–drug interactions. Which one of these can be considered to be a beneficial interaction and has been used therapeutically?**

☐ **A**   Cimetidine and dapsone

☐ **B**   Cimetidine and phenytoin

☐ **C**   Cisapride and erythromycin

☐ **D**   Rifampicin and ciclosporin A

☐ **E**   Ritonavir and fluoxetine

1.54   **Which one of the following statements relating to the use of acetylcholinesterase inhibitors in the treatment of Alzheimer's disease is true?**

☐ **A**   Donepezil binds to the esteratic site of the enzyme

☐ **B**   Donepezil has a half-life of 7 hours

☐ **C**   Metrifonate binds reversibly to the active site of the enzyme

☐ **D**   Rivastigmine binds to both the anionic and esteratic sites of the enzyme

☐ **E**   The metabolite of metrifonate does not possess any pharmacological activity

1.55   **Below is a list of drugs with their putative adverse reactions. Which one of the pairings is not correct?**

☐ **A**   Cerivastatin–rhabdomyolysis

☐ **B**   Indinavir–renal stones

☐ **C**   Pergolide–pulmonary fibrosis

☐ **D**   Tolcapone–neuroleptic malignant syndrome

☐ **E**   Vigabatrin–anterior uveitis

1.56 **Which one of the following statements about leflunomide is incorrect?**

☐ **A** It can be classed as a disease-modifying antirheumatic drug

☐ **B** It has active metabolites

☐ **C** It has comparable efficacy to sulfasalazine and methotrexate

☐ **D** It inhibits dihydro-orotate dehydrogenase

☐ **E** It inhibits purine synthesis

1.57 **During warfarin therapy which one of the following statements is correct?**

☐ **A** Dosage is adjusted by monitoring drug levels

☐ **B** Dose requirements are genetically determined

☐ **C** Osteoporosis may develop

☐ **D** Overdose can be reversed by protamine sulphate

☐ **E** Therapeutic effect is usually achieved within 24 hours

1.58 **When inducing local anaesthesia by infiltration, which one of the following is correct?**

☐ **A** Accidental injection of lidocaine (lignocaine) into the systemic circulation may increase myocardial and neuronal excitability

☐ **B** Bupivacaine produces a shorter-lasting anaesthesia than lidocaine

☐ **C** The anaesthetic agents used are strongly acidic

☐ **D** The duration of anaesthesia may be prolonged by the addition of salbutamol

☐ **E** The duration of anaesthesia with lidocaine depends on diffusion and not on drug metabolism

1.59 **Which one of the following statements regarding combined hormonal oral contraceptives is incorrect?**

☐ **A** Oestrogen preparations promote blood clotting

☐ **B** Oestrogens inhibit follicle stimulating hormone (FSH) release

☐ **C** Progestogens inhibit luteinising hormone (LH) release

☐ **D** The incidence of benign breast disease may be increased

☐ **E** The risk of stroke is increased to a small extent

Answers on pages 83–102

1.60   **In relation to the use of interferon-β in the treatment of multiple sclerosis, which one of the following is incorrect?**

☐   **A**   Does not have a beneficial effect if administered at the time of the first ever demyelinating event

☐   **B**   Reduces brain atrophy

☐   **C**   Reduces relapses in patients with chronic multiple sclerosis

☐   **D**   Reduces the development of brain lesions on magnetic resonance imaging (MRI)

☐   **E**   Slows progression of physical disability

Endocrinology

Best of Five

Questions

ENDOCRINOLOGY: 'BEST OF FIVE' QUESTIONS

For each of the questions select the ONE most appropriate answer from the options provided.

2.1   You are asked to review a 73-year-old woman who is drowsy and rather vague 4 days after abdominal surgery. The surgical house officer has done thyroid function tests which show: thyroid stimulating hormone (TSH) = 0.2 (normal range 0.4–4.0 mU/l); free T_3 = 2.1 (normal range 2.5–6.5 pmol/l); free T_4 = 22 (normal range 10–25 pmol/l). What is the most likely explanation for these test results?

☐ **A** Primary hypothyroidism

☐ **B** Secondary hypothyroidism

☐ **C** Sick euthyroidism

☐ **D** Drug interference

☐ **E** Laboratory error

2.2   A 28-year-old woman is noticed by her GP to have a lump in her neck, which moves on swallowing consistent with a thyroid nodule. Thyroid function tests are normal. On examination she has a 2–3 cm thyroid nodule with no neck lymph nodes. There is no family history of thyroid disease. What is the best course of action to advise?

☐ **A** No further investigation is necessary as she is euthyroid and the lesion is very likely to be benign

☐ **B** To have a radionucleotide thyroid scan to determine if the nodule is 'hot' or 'cold'

☐ **C** To have an ultrasound of the thyroid and if the nodule is partly cystic then no further treatment is necessary

☐ **D** To have a fine needle aspiration of the nodule for cytology

☐ **E** To have a 3-month trial of thyroxine and proceed to further investigation if the nodule fails to reduce in size

2.3 **A 53-year-old man without a previous diagnosis of diabetes is noted on a hospital admission for pneumonia to have a random glucose of 9.5 mmol/l. His GP repeats a fasting value on two occasions several weeks after discharge when he has recovered. The results are 6.4 and 6.7 mmol/l. Which of the following would be the most appropriate course of action?**

☐ **A** To reassure him that he does not have diabetes and advise no further action

☐ **B** To encourage him to pursue a diet and exercise programme

☐ **C** To register him for the regional retinopathy screening programme

☐ **D** To begin him on metformin

☐ **E** To begin him on gliclazide

2.4 **A 21-year-old man with type 1 diabetes since age 9 presents having had two fits in the night on separate occasions. His morning blood sugars vary from 2.5 mmol/l to 15 mmol/l. He currently takes soluble (humulin S) insulin before meals and isophane insulin (humulin I) at night-time. Which of the following would be the most appropriate next step?**

☐ **A** Begin treatment with sodium valproate pending other investigations

☐ **B** To reduce his pre-evening meal soluble insulin dose

☐ **C** To ask him to set his alarm clock for 0300 h to test his blood sugar on two occasions

☐ **D** To reduce his evening carbohydrate content

☐ **E** To request a computed tomography (CT) brain

2.5 **Which of the following is most appropriate regarding type 2 diabetes?**

☐ **A** 5–10% of patients will ultimately need treatment with insulin

☐ **B** Patients with hepatocyte nuclear factor (HNF)-1 alpha mutations causing maturity-onset diabetes of the young (MODY-3) can be very successfully treated with sulphonylurea drugs

☐ **C** Weight loss is able to prevent progression from impaired glucose tolerance to diabetes but cannot reverse established diabetes

☐ **D** Raised liver enzyme levels are not typical and should prompt a search for an unrelated cause

☐ **E** Hypercholesterolaemia is the typical lipid abnormality

Answers on pages 105–121

2.6 **Which of the following are true of Turner's syndrome?**

- ☐ **A** Aortic root rupture is an important cause of death
- ☐ **B** Growth hormone treatment for short stature is ineffective
- ☐ **C** The phenotype is only apparent in girls if one X chromosome is completely absent
- ☐ **D** Partial X chromosome deletion in boys can result in a similar phenotype
- ☐ **E** The phenotype is not apparent before the age of 1 year

2.7 **A 77-year-old man presenting with lethargy and drowsiness was noted to have a serum sodium of 123 mmol/l. Further investigations revealed $K^+ = 4.2$ mmol/l. Which of the following is most appropriate?**

- ☐ **A** Blood glucose should be measured as a markedly raised level may account for the hyponatraemia
- ☐ **B** If the serum osmolality is low, then hypertriglyceridaemia or paraproteinaemia are likely causes
- ☐ **C** If the urine sodium is low, syndrome of inappropriate antidiuretic hormone (ADH) secretion is a likely cause
- ☐ **D** Thyroid function tests should be requested to exclude hyperthyroidism
- ☐ **E** Hypoadrenalism is unlikely as the potassium is not raised

2.8 **A 42-year-old woman is noted to have potassium of 2.1 mmol/l on a routine preoperative assessment. She denies any regular medication. Which one of the following is most appropriate?**

- ☐ **A** Serum magnesium level should be measured to exclude Bartter's syndrome
- ☐ **B** The presence of hypertension would suggest Gittelman's syndrome
- ☐ **C** Renin–aldosterone testing should be performed even if the patient is normotensive
- ☐ **D** Excess liquorice consumption may be a cause if the patient is normotensive
- ☐ **E** Occult use of purgatives is a possible cause if the urine potassium is low

2.9 **Which of the following are true of hormone release from adipose tissue?**

☐ **A** Leptin increases appetite

☐ **B** Adiponectin results in increased insulin resistance

☐ **C** Leptin is important in the timing of puberty

☐ **D** Leptin deficiency is associated with low body weight

☐ **E** Serum leptin levels do not correlate with body weight

2.10 **A 15-year-old boy is concerned that he is the smallest in his class at school. Which of the following is most likely to be true/important?**

☐ **A** Constitutional delay of puberty is very unlikely at this age

☐ **B** The heights of both parents should be measured

☐ **C** If a systemic illness were causing delayed growth it would be apparent

☐ **D** A chromosomal analysis is mandatory

☐ **E** A hamartoma of the pineal is a classical cause

2.11 **Which of the following are true of insulin action?**

☐ **A** A significant portion of its action is mediated via cyclic AMP

☐ **B** Abnormalities in the insulin receptor are seen in up to 10% of patients with type 2 diabetes

☐ **C** The majority of abnormalities of insulin action in type 2 diabetes have now been characterised at the molecular level

☐ **D** The insulin receptor complex can acquire enzymatic function

☐ **E** The insulin receptor complex migrates into the nucleus once activated

2.12 **In the diagnosis of Cushing's syndrome, which of the following is true?**

☐ **A** Suppression of cortisol production in the high dose dexamethasone test suggests an adrenal adenoma

☐ **B** A normal adrenocorticotrophic hormone (ACTH) level excludes the diagnosis of pituitary-dependent Cushing's syndrome (Cushing's disease)

☐ **C** Sampling of ACTH from the draining venous plexus of the pituitary may be required

☐ **D** The CRH stimulation test is no longer used

☐ **E** A bronchial lesion causing ectopic ACTH secretion is usually apparent on chest X-ray

Answers on pages 105–121

2.13 **A 33-year-old lady with type 2 diabetes presents in early pregnancy. Which of the following is most appropriate?**

□ **A** She can continue metformin but needs to stop any sulphonylurea drugs she is taking

□ **B** She must convert onto insulin therapy

□ **C** She should continue her antihypertensive and lipid lowering medications during pregnancy

□ **D** The outcome of pregnancy is better than in type 1 diabetes

□ **E** If she has microalbuminuria but not a raised creatinine, this is unlikely to change during pregnancy

2.14 **In a patient with suspected acromegaly, which one of the following is true?**

□ **A** An increase in colonic polyps is an associated feature, but these are not premalignant

□ **B** A pituitary tumour can usually be seen on magnetic resonance imaging (MRI) scanning

□ **C** A raised fasting growth hormone (GH) level confirms the diagnosis

□ **D** A raised prolactin level makes the diagnosis unlikely

□ **E** Successful treatment results in resolution of the facial changes

2.15 **Which one of the following statements is most accurate concerning antidiuretic hormone (ADH)?**

□ **A** It circulates in the bloodstream bound to neurophysin

□ **B** It is a linear octapeptide

□ **C** It is released by ethanol

□ **D** It is synthesised in the hypothalamus

□ **E** Its release is inhibited by carbamazepine

2.16   **Which one of the following is commonly associated with a diagnosis of diabetes insipidus (DI)?**

☐   **A**   A requirement for urgent diagnosis and treatment with vasopressin in the central form (cranial diabetes insipidus) to avoid mortality

☐   **B**   A serum sodium of less than 130 mmol/l

☐   **C**   Autosomal dominant inheritance in the congenital nephrogenic form

☐   **D**   Lithium therapy

☐   **E**   Worsening with thiazide diuretics in the nephrogenic form

2.17   **A 23-year-old woman presents with galactorrhoea. Which one of the following is most important to consider in an investigation of this case?**

☐   **A**   A careful search for an underlying malignancy

☐   **B**   Exclusion of chronic liver disease

☐   **C**   Exclusion of treatment with antiemetic drugs

☐   **D**   Exclusion of treatment with tricyclic antidepressant drugs

☐   **E**   If associated with a prolactin level of < 5000 mU/l (normal range < 450 U/l) then a magnetic resonance imaging (MRI) scan of the pituitary is rarely necessary

2.18   **A 19-year-old woman with a body mass index (BMI) of 16.1 kg/m² is considered to have anorexia nervosa. Which one of the following is not consistent with this diagnosis alone?**

☐   **A**   Elevated luteinising hormone (LH) levels

☐   **B**   Loss of axillary hair

☐   **C**   Presentation with primary amenorrhoea

☐   **D**   Raised cortisol levels

☐   **E**   Raised growth hormone levels

Answers on pages 105–121

2.19 **Hypogonadism in a 20-year-old phenotypic man may be associated with which one of the following?**

☐ **A** Anosmia

☐ **B** Complete androgen resistance (testicular feminisation)

☐ **C** Exposure to androgens in utero

☐ **D** Low levels of sex hormone binding globulin

☐ **E** Low levels of luteinising hormone (LH) and follicle stimulating hormone (FSH) in association with the XXY karyotype

2.20 **A 33-year-old woman presents with hyperthyroidism and proptosis with diplopia and periorbital oedema. Which one of the following is most likely to be true?**

☐ **A** Antithyroid microsomal (antithyroid peroxidase) antibodies are likely to be present and responsible for stimulating the thyroid to overproduce thyroid hormone

☐ **B** If the woman becomes pregnant, transplacental passage of thyroxine may result in hyperthyroidism in the baby for several weeks (neonatal hyperthyroidism), even after the disease has been brought under control with antithyroid drugs

☐ **C** Levels of thyroid stimulating hormone (TSH) are likely to be in the normal range

☐ **D** Radioiodine may not be the ideal first line treatment

☐ **E** The eye signs are very likely to improve with treatment of her hyperthyroidism

2.21 **In a 45-year-old woman presenting with profound primary hypothyroidism due to autoimmune thyroiditis, which one of the following is unlikely to be linked to the diagnosis?**

☐ **A** Addison's disease

☐ **B** Ataxia

☐ **C** Cardiomyopathy

☐ **D** Paranoia and delusions

☐ **E** Thyroid lymphoma

Answers on pages 105–121

2.22 **Which one of the following suggests that thyrotoxicosis in a 28-year-old woman will resolve spontaneously and is best treated expectantly?**

☐ **A** Diarrhoea

☐ **B** Diffuse uptake on radioiodine scanning

☐ **C** Mild thyroid eye disease

☐ **D** Patchy uptake on radioiodine scanning

☐ **E** Tenderness over the thyroid gland

2.23 **A 33-year-old woman presenting with palpitations is found to have a thyroid stimulating hormone (TSH) level of < 0.1 mU/l and a free T_4 of 31 pmol/l (normal range 10–24). Which one of the following might best explain this pattern?**

☐ **A** Amiodarone therapy

☐ **B** Late pregnancy

☐ **C** Occult abuse of T_3

☐ **D** Systemic illness such as pneumonia

☐ **E** Treatment with the oral contraceptive

2.24 **A G-protein mutation may result in which one of the following?**

☐ **A** A non-functioning pituitary tumour

☐ **B** Multiple endocrine neoplasia type 2 syndrome

☐ **C** Persistent generation of cyclic adenosine monophosphate (AMP)

☐ **D** Persistent hydrolysis of ATP

☐ **E** Hypercalcaemia

Answers on pages 105–121

2.25   A 32-year-old woman presents with rapidly progressive hirsutism over the last 4 months, weight gain and muscle weakness. On examination she has clitoromegaly and a 'moon face'. Investigations reveal a raised 24-hour urinary free cortisol and an undetectable level of adrenocorticotrophic hormone (ACTH) on two occasions. Which one of the following is the most likely underlying diagnosis?

☐ **A** An adrenal adenoma
☐ **B** An adrenal carcinoma
☐ **C** A bronchial carcinoid
☐ **D** A bronchial carcinoma
☐ **E** A pituitary tumour

2.26   Which one of the following is true of atrial natriuretic peptide?

☐ **A** It causes increased thirst
☐ **B** It causes salt craving
☐ **C** It causes vasodilatation
☐ **D** It is secreted by the juxtaglomerular apparatus
☐ **E** It suppresses the release of aldosterone

2.27   Which one of the following features is the best early indicator of inadequate glucocorticoid replacement in patients with adrenal failure?

☐ **A** Fatigue
☐ **B** Hypoglycaemia
☐ **C** Hyperkalaemia
☐ **D** Hypokalaemia
☐ **E** Salt craving

2.28   In an infant with homozygous congenital adrenal hyperplasia due to 21-hydroxylase deficiency, which one of the following is most likely?

☐ **A** A female infant will present with intersex
☐ **B** A male infant will be feminised
☐ **C** Hypertension will develop in the first year
☐ **D** No effect will be apparent until puberty
☐ **E** 17-OH progesterone levels will be low

2.29 **Idiopathic hypoparathyroidism is most frequently associated with which one of the following?**

☐ **A** A good response in terms of calcium levels to treatment with calcium and vitamin D

☐ **B** Calcification of the tympanic membranes

☐ **C** Characteristic facies

☐ **D** Hyperthyroidism

☐ **E** Short fourth and fifth metacarpals

2.30 **With regard to Paget's disease, which one of the following statements is most true?**

☐ **A** Asymptomatic disease should be treated aggressively

☐ **B** Patients respond well to ergocalciferol

☐ **C** Serum alkaline phosphatase reflects disease activity

☐ **D** The disease is primarily a disorder of bone mineralisation

☐ **E** The number of lesions normally increases over time

2.31 **Features of multiple endocrine neoplasia (MEN) type 1 include which one of the following?**

☐ **A** Adrenal nodules

☐ **B** Hyperparathyroidism

☐ **C** Hyperthyroidism

☐ **D** Hypothyroidism

☐ **E** Phaeochromocytoma

2.32 **Which one of the following elements is most important in investigation of spontaneous fasting hypoglycaemia?**

☐ **A** A sulphonylurea screen

☐ **B** Magnetic resonance imaging (MRI) of the adrenals

☐ **C** MRI of the pituitary

☐ **D** Thyroid function

☐ **E** 24-hour urinary free cortisol

Answers on pages 105–121

2.33 **Which one of the following is of most value in the management of phaeochromocytoma?**

☐ **A** Early treatment with β-blockade

☐ **B** Exclusion of associated islet cell tumours

☐ **C** Radiotherapy in the management of malignant disease

☐ **D** Surgical histology as an indicator of malignancy

☐ **E** Yearly screening with urinary catecholamines in familial disease

2.34 **Which one of the following statements is true?**

☐ **A** Carbamazepine lowers vasopressin levels

☐ **B** Desmopressin acetate has vasoconstrictive effects

☐ **C** High gastrin levels are associated with pernicious anaemia

☐ **D** In the absence of calcitonin, calcium levels rise

☐ **E** The glucagon response to hypoglycaemia is exaggerated in longstanding type 1 diabetes

2.35 **A 29-year-old primigravida woman with hyperemesis at 9 weeks of pregnancy has her thyroid function tests measured because of a resting tachycardia. These show thyroid stimulating hormone (TSH) < 0.1 mU/l (normal range 0.4–4.5), free T_3 6.8 pmol/l (normal range 2.5–5.2). There is no previous history of thyroid disease. On examination she has minimal non-tender thyroid enlargement. Ultrasound reveals a single live conceptus. Which one of the following is the most appropriate management strategy?**

☐ **A** Advise termination of pregnancy

☐ **B** Commence treatment immediately with propylthiouracil with a view to dose adjustments through the remainder of pregnancy

☐ **C** Commence treatment immediately with propylthiouracil with a view to performing subtotal thyroidectomy in the second trimester of pregnancy

☐ **D** Withhold any antithyroid treatment and repeat thyroid function testing in 3 weeks

☐ **E** Withhold any antithyroid treatment pending a radionucleotide thyroid scan to exclude transient thyroiditis

2.36   A 54-year-old man who has had trans-sphenoidal surgery and external beam radiotherapy for a non-functioning pituitary tumour 6 years previously has been seen by his GP recently, feeling increasingly tired with loss of libido. Tests done at that consultation showed testosterone < 0.1 nmol/l (normal range 10–30), thyroid stimulating hormone (TSH) 2.3 mU/l. He now presents to the Emergency Department with vomiting. Blood pressure (BP) is 90/60 mmHg, sodium 121 mmol/l, potassium 3.8 mmol/l. He is on no medication. Which one of the following is the most appropriate immediate course of action?

    ☐ **A** Admit the patient for an insulin stress test to assess pituitary function

    ☐ **B** Immediate treatment with intramuscular testosterone

    ☐ **C** Immediate treatment with thyroxine

    ☐ **D** Rehydrate with saline and then arrange a short Synacthen test

    ☐ **E** Short Synacthen testing followed by immediate treatment with hydrocortisone

2.37   In the treatment of an acute asthmatic attack, β-agonists and corticosteroids are frequently used. Which one of the following is true of the molecular mechanism by which these agents act?

    ☐ **A** β-agonists have a prolonged action because they act by both modulating gene transcription and an intracellular second messenger

    ☐ **B** Both agents act quickly because they act via an intracellular second messenger

    ☐ **C** Both agents act quickly because they have specific cellular receptors

    ☐ **D** Corticosteroids act more slowly because they act by modulating gene transcription

    ☐ **E** Corticosteroids have a prolonged action because they are lipid soluble

2.38   In a hypertensive individual, which one of the following is the likely finding in a patient with renal artery stenosis and is helpful in distinguishing the condition from Conn's syndrome?

    ☐ **A** A high aldosterone level

    ☐ **B** A high renin and a high aldosterone level

    ☐ **C** A high renin level and a low aldosterone level

    ☐ **D** A low aldosterone level

    ☐ **E** A low renin and a high aldosterone level

2.39 An overweight 43-year-old woman is referred with the clinical appearance of Cushing's syndrome and a blood pressure of 170/90 mmHg. The most convenient initial test to distinguish this diagnosis from simple obesity would be?

☐ **A** An adrenocorticotrophic hormone (ACTH) level

☐ **B** An adrenal magnetic resonance imaging (MRI) scan

☐ **C** A midnight salivary cortisol level

☐ **D** Serum potassium and bicarbonate

☐ **E** 24-hour urinary free cortisol

2.40 A 60-year-old gentleman with type 2 diabetes has a myocardial infarction. He is treated initially with an intravenous infusion of insulin. He has an episode of left ventricular failure and is started on an angiotensin-converting enzyme (ACE) inhibitor. He has a degree of renal dysfunction with a creatinine of 147 µmol/l, which is stable. He is usually on 80 mg bd of gliclazide. You notice that his haemoglobin Hb A_{1c} is 11.2% and on dietician review there is not much that can be changed. Which one of the following is the most appropriate therapy for his diabetes?

☐ **A** Acarbose

☐ **B** Basal bolus insulin

☐ **C** Increase gliclazide to 160 mg bd

☐ **D** Metformin

☐ **E** Rosiglitazone

2.41 A 32-year-old man who has had type 1 diabetes for 12 years reports episodes of confusion occurring without warning. On one of these occasions, the blood sugar level on home testing was 2.5 mmol/l. The single best advice to help this patient for the future would be?

☐ **A** To eat every 2 hours

☐ **B** To eat less carbohydrate with each meal

☐ **C** To increase his insulin at night and reduce it during the day for 3 months

☐ **D** To reduce his insulin to maintain relatively high blood sugars (8–15 mmol/l) for at least 3 months

☐ **E** To test his blood sugar a minimum of four times daily every day

2.42 **In a patient with diabetes and microalbuminuria, the most important element of management to preserve renal function is?**

- ☐ **A** Aggressive management of hyperlipidaemia
- ☐ **B** Aggressive management of hypertension
- ☐ **C** A low protein diet
- ☐ **D** Avoidance of diuretic use
- ☐ **E** Improvement of glycaemic control

2.43 **In a 52-year-old man with acromegaly and a moderately sized (1.5 cm) pituitary tumour, the most appropriate first line of therapy would be?**

- ☐ **A** Bromocriptine therapy
- ☐ **B** External beam radiotherapy
- ☐ **C** Octreotide therapy
- ☐ **D** Trans-sphenoidal surgery
- ☐ **E** Yttrium implants into the pituitary

2.44 **Appropriate hormone replacement medication for a 28-year-old woman with primary adrenocortical failure (Addison's disease) would be?**

- ☐ **A** Dexamethasone 0.5 mg daily alone
- ☐ **B** Hydrocortisone 10 mg mane and fludrocortisone 100 μg mane
- ☐ **C** Hydrocortisone 10 mg mane and 5 mg pm, and fludrocortisone 100 μg mane
- ☐ **D** Hydrocortisone 50 mg bd and fludrocortisone 100 μg mane
- ☐ **E** Prednisolone 15 mg mane and fludrocortisone 100 μg mane

2.45 **In an individual known to have the genetic mutation responsible for multiple endocrine neoplasia type 2, which one of the following describes the two most important elements in management?**

- ☐ **A** Prophylactic thyroidectomy and bilateral adrenalectomy
- ☐ **B** Prophylactic thyroidectomy and regular pituitary imaging
- ☐ **C** Prophylactic thyroidectomy and regular screening for phaeochromocytoma
- ☐ **D** Regular thyroid imaging and regular screening for phaeochromocytoma
- ☐ **E** Regular thyroid and pituitary imaging

Answers on pages 105–121

2.46 **A 23-year-old woman presents concerned about increased hair growth. She is noted to have dark facial and lower abdominal hairs. She menstruates regularly but her cycle length varies from 3 to 6 weeks. Which one of the following is correct?**

☐ **A** A benign course is very likely in such cases

☐ **B** Clitoromegaly is frequently observed in such cases

☐ **C** If the diagnosis were polycystic ovarian syndrome, recent onset of hair growth would be expected

☐ **D** Radiological imaging for a tumour of the ovary should routinely be performed in all such cases

☐ **E** Testosterone levels would be expected in the low–normal male range in such cases

2.47 **A 39-year-old man presents with a 2-week history of polydipsia and polyuria. He is found to have a random glucose of 17.3 mmol/l. There are no ketones in the urine. He denies recent weight loss or vomiting. His body mass index (BMI) is 24.7 kg/m². Which one of the following is correct?**

☐ **A** He could be started on a sulphonylurea, taught to test his own capillary glucose levels and be reassessed in 1 month

☐ **B** As in A but review in 3 months is more appropriate to assess progress

☐ **C** He should be admitted to hospital urgently to commence insulin therapy

☐ **D** He should be referred to a dietitian and reviewed after three months of diet and exercise therapy

☐ **E** The optimal therapy is metformin

2.48 **Which one of the following is true regarding carbohydrate metabolism after 48 hours of fasting?**

☐ **A** Amino acids are an increasingly important source of substrates for glucose synthesis

☐ **B** Fatty acids provide 15–20% of the substrates for glucose synthesis

☐ **C** Glucagon levels are rising

☐ **D** Ketonuria is rare

☐ **E** Liver glycogen is an important source of glucose

2.49   A 23-year-old man is found on routine screening to have a cholesterol level of 11.3 mmol/l, a triglyceride level of 1.2 mmol/l and a high density lipoprotein (HDL) level of 1.1 mmol/l. His mother died aged 45 of a heart attack. Which one of the following is most appropriate in this case?

☐   **A**   Excess alcohol is a possible cause

☐   **B**   He should have a 3-month trial of dietary advice before commencing lipid-lowering therapy

☐   **C**   Treatment should commence with a fibrate

☐   **D**   Treatment should commence with a statin

☐   **E**   Undiagnosed diabetes mellitus is a likely cause

2.50   A 64-year-old lady is noted to have a corrected calcium level of 2.85 mmol/l during blood testing for 'tiredness'. Which one of the following statements is most appropriate in this case?

☐   **A**   A parathyroid hormone level in the high–normal range makes hyperparathyroidism unlikely

☐   **B**   A raised alkaline phosphatase level suggests bony metastases

☐   **C**   Hyperparathyroidism and malignancy account for 90% of cases

☐   **D**   If it is due to hyperparathyroidism, parathyroidectomy is invariably required

☐   **E**   If the patient is asymptomatic, no further investigation is required

Gastroenterology

Best of Five

Questions

GASTROENTEROLOGY: 'BEST OF FIVE' QUESTIONS

For each of the questions select the ONE most appropriate answer from the options provided.

3.1   A pregnant Taiwanese woman has routine hepatitis screening and is found to be hepatitis B surface antigen positive. Subsequent testing reveals that she is e antigen negative and has a low viral load (<10^5 copies/ml). Which of the following is correct?

☐   **A**   The child is at no risk of developing chronic hepatitis B

☐   **B**   The child should be treated with hepatitis B immunoglobulin (HBIG) after birth

☐   **C**   The mother should be discouraged from breast-feeding

☐   **D**   The mother has most likely acquired her hepatitis during pregnancy

☐   **E**   The child should be offered vaccination against hepatitis B as soon as possible after birth

3.2   A 54-year-old woman is referred with a history of pruritus and lethargy that dates back many months. She has abnormal liver function tests, total bilirubin 26 μmol/l, alanine aminotransferase (ALT) 40 U/l, alkaline phosphate 412 U/l, albumin 36 g/l and a fasting cholesterol 7.6 mmol/l. An abdominal ultrasound scan shows no evidence of bile duct obstruction or obvious liver disease. Subsequently, you find she has a positive antimitochondrial antibody result. Her liver biopsy histology shows periportal fibrosis and inflammation. You tell her that she has primary biliary cirrhosis. Which one of the following is most accurate?

☐   **A**   As the pruritus is due to raised circulating bilirubin levels, bile salt binding agents such as colestyramine are likely to give symptom relief

☐   **B**   Because primary biliary cirrhosis is an autoimmune disease, oral steroids are likely to be helpful

☐   **C**   She has a high risk of atherosclerosis

☐   **D**   Antimitochondrial antibodies can be used to assess treatment response

☐   **E**   Ursodeoxycholic acid will help her symptoms and may delay disease progression

3.3   A young woman is brought into hospital as an emergency by ambulance.
        She had been found, drowsy, by her boyfriend on his return home from
        work that evening. He tells you that they had had a row that morning. He
        had found an empty packet of paracetamol tablets in the kitchen. You
        make a rapid clinical assessment of the patient and note her stable
        observations but depressed Glasgow Coma Scale score of 13/15. You
        obtain a venous blood sample to send to the laboratory for tests. Which
        one of the following would be your next priority?

  □ **A** Arrange urgent gastric lavage
  □ **B** Ask the nursing staff to monitor her blood glucose levels
  □ **C** Contact your regional liver unit as the patient has clearly taken a
          significant overdose and may need transfer
  □ **D** Seek psychiatric input
  □ **E** Start an *N*-acetylcysteine infusion

3.4   A retired man presents with tingling in his hands and feet. He admits to
        having a poor appetite and modest weight loss over the past year though
        you find it difficult to keep him focused on the consultation. On clinical
        examination you are struck by his pallor and the beefy appearance of his
        tongue. He also appears to have paraesthesiae in a 'glove and stocking'
        distribution and muscle wasting. You are not surprised to find a
        macrocytosis on his blood film. Which is the most likely explanation for
        his presentation?

  □ **A** Chronic pancreatitis
  □ **B** Coeliac disease
  □ **C** His use of over-the-counter vitamin C preparations
  □ **D** Inadequate diet
  □ **E** Pernicious anaemia

Answers on pages 125–142

3.5   The report from your patient's recent elective oesophagogastroduodenoscopy comments on an incidental finding of prominent oesophageal varices. In addition to the need to determine the cause for the varices, further management should include which one of the following?

☐ **A** No treatment is required unless there has been an index variceal bleed

☐ **B** Serial endoscopy and variceal sclerotherapy until the varices have been eradicated

☐ **C** The regular use of a vasopressin analogue such as terlipressin to maintain portal pressure below 12 mmHg

☐ **D** The use of a non-selective β-blocker such as propranolol to maintain portal pressure below 12 mmHg

☐ **E** The use of a selective β-blocker such as atenolol to maintain portal pressure below 15 mmHg

3.6   A 65-year-old man recovering from chemotherapy for lymphoma is admitted to hospital with malnourishment secondary to painful stomatitis. He is assessed and found to be 50 kg with a BMI of 17 kg/m^2. Looking back through his medical records his weight is documented at 57 kg 2 months previously. Which of the following is true?

☐ **A** Total energy intake should be 25–35 kcal/kg per day

☐ **B** Parenteral nutrition should be instigated immediately

☐ **C** Nasogastric feeding will be unhelpful

☐ **D** Serum Potassium monitoring is essential

☐ **E** Thiamine and vitamin B replacement will not be required

3.7   Acquired immunodeficiency may be associated with several gastrointestinal and liver disorders. Which one of the following would be least likely to be associated with advanced HIV infection?

☐ **A** Anal tumours

☐ **B** Chronic hepatitis C infection

☐ **C** *Cryptosporidium*-associated diarrhoea

☐ **D** Hepatitis B surface antigen-positive status

☐ **E** Troublesome perianal Crohn's disease

3.8   **A 21-year-old student emails her GP from a backpacking trip around South America with a 2-week history of watery stools. She is concerned about a long train journey she must make the following day. There is no blood in the stool but she feels light-headed and faint. Which of the following is correct?**

☐ **A**   The commonest cause of travellers' diarrhoea is *Campylobacter*

☐ **B**   A useful rehydration solution can be made using 8 level teaspoons of sugar and 8 level teaspoons of salt in 1 litre of water

☐ **C**   A single dose of ciprofloxacin may be of benefit

☐ **D**   If her diarrhoea persists for longer than 4 weeks it cannot be travellers' diarrhoea

☐ **E**   South America is the continent responsible for the most cases of travellers' diarrhoea in UK travellers

3.9   **You have invited a friend with coeliac disease round for dinner. You have decided what you are going to eat and drink. You have taken care to remove pasta and cakes from the menu, but then realise that you may be drinking alone. Which one of the following had you planned to serve?**

☐ **A**   A low-alcohol lager

☐ **B**   Cranberry juice

☐ **C**   Gin and tonic

☐ **D**   Green tea

☐ **E** ´ White wine

Answers on pages 125–142

3.10   Every week a district nurse has been visiting an 80-year-old woman at
        home to dress chronic leg ulcers. Two weeks ago he had felt that the
        ulcers had become infected. In consultation with the patient's GP he has
        decided to start treatment with the antibiotic metronidazole. He was
        unable to visit last week, but on his return earlier today he discovered
        that the woman had developed the most appalling diarrhoea. The patient
        had also become somewhat confused. She appeared dehydrated, pulse
        86 bpm and temperature 37.6 °C. The nurse observed traces of bright
        blood in the toilet. What advice would you give to him?

☐   A   It would be reasonable to stop the antibiotic, give Dioralyte (an oral
        rehydration salt) and review the patient in 72 hours

☐   B   She must be sent to hospital as she is confused

☐   C   She must be sent to hospital as she is dehydrated and pyrexial: given
        the history you are concerned to diagnose and treat any antibiotic
        associated complications as soon as possible

☐   D   She must be sent to hospital for further assessment as she is dehydrated
        and pyrexial, although pseudomembranous colitis can be discounted
        as the cause, as metronidazole is used as treatment for this condition –
        it does not cause it

☐   E   You feel that ischaemic colitis seems most likely given her chronic leg
        ulceration. In addition, your records show that she has been an in-
        patient recently and was successfully treated for *Clostridium difficile*-
        associated colitis. Relapse is very uncommon after treatment

3.11   A 72-year-old woman presents to the Out-patients' Department with a
        2-month history of significant weight loss, severe and constant back ache
        and a 2-week history of jaundice. Her past medical history includes atrial
        fibrillation and diabetes diagnosed 6 months previously. An urgent
        ultrasound scan reveals no evidence of gallstones but a dilated biliary
        system and a mass in the head of the pancreas. A presumptive diagnosis
        of pancreatic cancer is made. Which of the following is correct?

☐   A   Percutaneous biopsy should be taken for a tissue diagnosis before
        possible surgery

☐   B   The persistent back ache is a poor prognostic sign

☐   C   If tumour resection is impossible palliative chemotherapy is ineffective

☐   D   Her past medical history is not relevant to her current problem

☐   E   If the tumour is unresectable a coeliac plexus block is unlikely to be of
        benefit

3.12 **A 32-year-old woman attends your surgery to discuss her dietary needs ahead of a planned pregnancy. She is concerned that, as she has had surgery for small bowel Crohn's disease some years ago, the general advice offered about folic acid supplementation may not be appropriate for her. Unfortunately, your records do not confirm what operation was performed. Which of the following is most accurate?**

☐ **A** As signs and symptoms of folate deficiency typically take 4 months to manifest themselves, and if her serum and red cell folate levels are satisfactory ahead of conception, she need not worry about taking folate supplements. The risk to the fetus of developing neural tube problems arises only in the first trimester of pregnancy

☐ **B** If her operation for Crohn's disease has left her with a blind loop, bacteria may be competing for her dietary folate so supplementation at a higher than normal dose may be sensible

☐ **C** If she has had her small bowel resected she may be malabsorbing folic acid and so supplementation at a higher than normal dose would be advised

☐ **D** She may follow normal advice on supplementation (folic acid 400 mg daily) but should also cook her food thoroughly to improve the bioavailability of dietary folate

☐ **E** She should ensure that her diet is rich in foods that contain folate, such as nuts, liver and green vegetables

3.13 **A 60-year-old executive presents with confusion. You had met him some months previously when he had ascites. A diagnosis of alcohol-induced cirrhotic liver disease was made. On this occasion you note stigmata of chronic liver disease, including spider naevi and mild gynaecomastia. You find no ascites but mild peripheral oedema. His blood profile shows a mild hyponatraemia (perhaps a consequence of the diuretics which you had started him on), a serum albumin of 22 g/l and liver function tests show an international normalised ratio (INR) of 2.1. Your view that his confusion reflects a hepatic encephalopathy is supported by which one of the following?**

☐ **A** An absent pupillary response

☐ **B** An associated headache

☐ **C** His family's description of an inversion of his normal sleep pattern

☐ **D** His inability to recall either the name of the Queen or the Prime Minister

☐ **E** Your clinical finding of hyporeflexia

3.14   A 29-year-old woman presents with an incidental finding of mild iron deficiency anaemia. Menstruation-associated blood loss, dietary insufficiency and malabsorption have been excluded by others. Indeed, the latter would have been very surprising, as you understand that she suffers from constipation rather than diarrhoea. She also admits to bright-red rectal bleeding and has been putting on weight. At flexible sigmoidoscopy you only find a discrete area of ulcerated anterior rectal mucosa. You take biopsies from the area but meanwhile you should do which one of the following?

    ☐   **A**   Consider that your findings are not adequate to explain her anaemia

    ☐   **B**   Express surprise at finding what appears to be a solitary rectal ulcer in a young woman

    ☐   **C**   Express surprise that the ulcer is sited anteriorly

    ☐   **D**   Offer advice on laxatives

    ☐   **E**   Offer to start the patient on mesalazine suppositories

3.15   A 35-year-old woman is found to have low haemoglobin and subsequent studies show that she has a low mean corpuscular volume (MCV) and serum ferritin, confirming iron deficiency anaemia. She is asymptomatic, eats a healthy diet and up until this month was a regular blood donor. Which of the following is correct?

    ☐   **A**   She should have a gastroscopy and colonoscopy (or barium enema)

    ☐   **B**   Blood donation cannot be the cause of her anaemia

    ☐   **C**   Urine dipstick is unlikely to aid diagnosis

    ☐   **D**   Coeliac serology should be checked

    ☐   **E**   Gastrointestinal (GI) malignancy is a likely cause of her anaemia

3.16   A 35-year-old man presents to his GP with a 2-month history of epigastric pain worse on eating curry and partially relieved by simple antacids. Which of the following is correct?

    ☐   **A**   He requires an upper gastrointestinal (GI) endoscopy

    ☐   **B**   He should be commenced on lifelong proton pump inhibitor (PPI) treatment

    ☐   **C**   He should be treated for *Helicobacter pylori*

    ☐   **D**   Lifestyle advice and simple antacids are unlikely to be effective

    ☐   **E**   He should be screened for anaemia

3.17   A 19-year-old Scottish man is found on routine screening to have a mildly raised alanine aminotransferase (ALT). A thorough clinical examination reveals no abnormality. He has blood tests in a hepatology clinic to screen for liver disease and is found to have a serum ceruloplasmin just below the normal range and a presumptive diagnosis of Wilson's disease is made. Which of the following is correct?

☐   **A**   An absence of Kayser–Fleischer rings on slit lamp examination will exclude a diagnosis of Wilson's disease

☐   **B**   The low ceruloplasmin is diagnostic of Wilson's disease

☐   **C**   Genetic testing is the easiest way to confirm diagnosis

☐   **D**   He requires a liver biopsy

☐   **E**   A low copper diet may be enough to treat mild disease

3.18   A 34-year-old man is referred by his GP after becoming mildly jaundiced on two occasions associated with flu-like symptoms. He is otherwise well and a screen for viral hepatitis is negative as is a monospot test. His other liver enzymes and full blood count are normal and there is nothing to find on examination. Which of the following is correct?

☐   **A**   The bilirubin is likely to be conjugated

☐   **B**   Gilbert's disease is unlikely, as the patient has associated symptoms

☐   **C**   He may have a genetic polymorphism on chromosome 2

☐   **D**   His bilirubin levels are likely to be >100 μmol/l

☐   **E**   A normal full blood count excludes a haemolytic process

3.19   A 60-year-old man is referred with abnormal liver function tests (raised alanine aminotransferase (ALT) and alkaline phosphatase). He has drunk 35 units of alcohol each week for the last 20 years. An ultrasound test shows a slightly irregular liver outline. Viral hepatitis and autoimmune serology are negative. A serum ferritin is reported as 800 μg/l. Which of the following is true?

☐   **A**   Genetic testing may aid diagnosis

☐   **B**   A liver biopsy will not be required

☐   **C**   Total body iron stores are unlikely to be more than 3 g

☐   **D**   Venesection will be required

☐   **E**   C282Y heterozygosity excludes a diagnosis of genetic haemochromatosis

3.20   **A 24-year-old man is admitted to hospital with a 24-hour history of vomiting and severe abdominal pain radiating to his back. He is tender in the epigastric and periumbilical region on examination and biochemistry reveals a serum amylase at four times the upper limit of normal. An ultrasound reveals no obvious abnormality and no gallstones. A provisional diagnosis of acute pancreatitis is made. Which of the following statements is correct?**

☐   **A**   There is overwhelming evidence that intravenous antibiotics are of benefit

☐   **B**   Plain abdominal films will be useful to aid diagnosis

☐   **C**   A cause for pancreatitis cannot be found in 50% of cases

☐   **D**   A C-reactive protein (CRP) > 150 mg/l at 48 hours is a poor prognostic indicator

☐   **E**   A low body mass index (BMI) is associated with a worse outcome

3.21   **A 32-year-old pilot presents with pain and difficulty on swallowing. Her GP, who had recently diagnosed Raynaud's phenomenon and started her on the calcium channel blocker nifedipine, postulates that the dysphagia may be stress-related as her fitness to fly was due for review. A trial of proton pump inhibitors (PPIs) has not really helped. Which one of the following statements offers the most appropriate action?**

☐   **A**   You agree with the GP and reassure the patient accordingly

☐   **B**   You arrange upper gastrointestinal (GI) tract endoscopy

☐   **C**   You consider that a trial period off nifedipine would help as that drug relaxes smooth muscle and so may interfere with oesophageal motility

☐   **D**   You suggest she sees a psychologist

☐   **E**   You wonder about calcinosis cutis, Raynaud's phenomenon, oesophageal dysfunction, sclerodactyly and telangiectasia (CREST) syndrome and so arrange oesophageal physiology studies

3.22   A 38-year-old man is referred by his GP with a history of intermittent
abdominal pain and episodes of facial flushing. Upper gastrointestinal
(GI) endoscopy is performed and a small ulcerating tumour is seen in the
third part of the duodenum. Biopsies of this lesion are reported as
showing features typical of a neuroendocrine tumour. Which of the
following statements is true?

- ☐ **A**   Liver metastases are unlikely
- ☐ **B**   A labelled octreotide scan will be unhelpful
- ☐ **C**   General anaesthesia should be avoided if possible
- ☐ **D**   Chromogranin A levels are likely to be normal
- ☐ **E**   There is a high chance of a diagnosis of MEN1

3.23   A 23-year-old man with recently diagnosed ulcerative colitis has been
brought into remission with steroids and is now ready for maintenance
therapy. Which of the following statements is true?

- ☐ **A**   Budesonide is a good choice due to lack of systemic steroid side-
effects
- ☐ **B**   Mesalazine has more side-effects than sulfasalazine
- ☐ **C**   He will require lifelong therapy
- ☐ **D**   Azathioprine has no role in the maintenance therapy of ulcerative
colitis
- ☐ **E**   Maintenance therapy may reduce the risk of colon cancer

3.24   A 56-year-old woman is seen in a follow-up clinic after a partial
gastrectomy for the removal of a small gastrointestinal stromal tumour
(GIST). The tumour has been classified histologically as very low risk of
malignancy but she is symptomatic with abdominal pain and bloating
after eating followed a couple of hours later by sweating and
palpitations. Which of the following is true?

- ☐ **A**   An insulinoma has been misdiagnosed as a GIST
- ☐ **B**   Bacterial overgrowth is likely to be responsible
- ☐ **C**   Acarbose might be of use in symptomatic control
- ☐ **D**   Recurrence of her GIST is likely
- ☐ **E**   Prokinetic agents will relieve her symptoms

    Answers on pages 125–142

3.25 The local Director of Public Health is investigating a suspected outbreak of food poisoning. Although no organism has been identified, he hopes that by taking a detailed history from each sufferer he may be able to identify the cause and source. Which one of the following statements is true?

- [ ] **A** Bloody diarrhoea that started within 6 hours suggests *Entamoeba histolytica*
- [ ] **B** If contaminated canned foods were the putative source, *Vibrio parahaemolyticus* is suggested
- [ ] **C** If only previously fit and healthy individuals were affected, *Escherichia coli* is likely to be the source
- [ ] **D** If rice was the putative contaminated food a *Campylobacter* species is likely
- [ ] **E** Symptoms of vomiting within 4 hours and diarrhoea within 10 hours suggest *Bacillus cereus* as a likely cause

3.26 A 35-year-old man with a long history of poorly controlled ulcerative colitis underwent panproctocolectomy 3 years ago. He has recently complained of an unexplained episode of fever and investigations show: bilirubin 35 µmol/l, albumin 35 g/l, alkaline phosphatase 400 U/l, alanine transaminase 50 U/l, antineutrophil cytoplasmic antibody (ANCA) +, antimitochondrial antibody −. An ultrasound of the liver shows no gallstones or bile duct dilatation. Which one of the following is the most likely explanation for the abnormal liver function tests?

- [ ] **A** Acute hepatitis A
- [ ] **B** Bile duct damage at the time of colectomy
- [ ] **C** Metastases from colorectal cancer
- [ ] **D** Primary biliary cirrhosis
- [ ] **E** Primary sclerosing cholangitis

3.27 **A 40-year-old man with Crohn's disease is admitted with weight loss and diarrhoea. On reviewing his symptoms he describes his stools as pale and runny. He recalls colicky abdominal pain and bloating. He is anaemic and his albumin is very low, although his C-reactive protein (CRP) and plasma viscosity were both normal. Which one of the following is the explanation for his symptoms?**

☐ **A** Acquired lactose intolerance

☐ **B** Active small bowel Crohn's disease

☐ **C** Bacterial overgrowth secondary to an enterocolic fistula

☐ **D** Bile salt diarrhoea

☐ **E** Small bowel strictures

3.28 **A 36-year-old woman presented for investigation of infertility. She had had scanty periods for 3 years, but was noted to be anaemic. Her weight had fallen progressively. She also experienced cramp, particularly in the hands. Other than pallor, angular stomatitis and oral aphthous ulcers, there was little to find on examination. Which one of the following is the most likely diagnosis?**

☐ **A** Coeliac disease

☐ **B** Crohn's disease

☐ **C** Giardiasis

☐ **D** Irritable bowel syndrome

☐ **E** Scleroderma

  Answers on pages 125–142

3.29   A 38-year-old woman is admitted as an emergency with massive
        haematemesis. She is teetotal and has no risk factors for chronic liver
        disease. She has no past medical history and has been asymptomatic
        apart from occasional vague abdominal pain. She is resuscitated in the
        emergency department and has an upper gastrointestinal (GI) endoscopy.
        A 5 cm submucosal tumour is noted in the fundus of the stomach that has
        ulcerated into the lumen and has caused a large amount of bleeding, and
        biopsies of the region taken during endoscopy show ulcerated mucosa
        only. These findings are felt by the endoscopist to be typical features of a
        gastrointestinal stromal tumour (GIST). Which of the following
        statements is true?

   □ **A**   The tumour is likely to be benign in nature
   □ **B**   Treatment with Glivec (Imatinib) may be necessary
   □ **C**   Percutaneous biopsy of the lesion should be performed to obtain a
              tissue diagnosis
   □ **D**   The size of the tumour is unimportant
   □ **E**   Bleeding is uncommon in this type of tumour

3.30   A 55-year-old man is referred for the investigation of iron deficiency
        anaemia. He eats a normal diet and has not lost blood from anywhere.
        There is no family history and no abnormal signs of examination, other
        than those of anaemia. Proctoscopy is normal. Which one of the
        following would be your initial investigation in this patient?

   □ **A**   Barium enema
   □ **B**   Barium meal
   □ **C**   Endoscopy
   □ **D**   Red cell scan
   □ **E**   Stool testing for occult bleeding

3.31 A 26-year-old woman presents with a 6-month history of colicky lower abdominal pain associated with loose stool. The stool is accompanied by mucus but not blood. Despite urgency she has noted incomplete evacuation and the need to strain during defecation. Her weight is increasing. During the last 12 months, she has moved house and then lost her job through redundancy. Bearing in mind the most likely diagnosis, what would you do next?

- ☐ **A** Arrange a barium enema
- ☐ **B** Arrange a colonoscopy
- ☐ **C** Reassure her with explanation of the diagnosis, without further investigation
- ☐ **D** Refer to a dietitian
- ☐ **E** Refer to a debt counsellor

3.32 A 26-year-old woman has a history of Crohn's disease, which has been extensively investigated and shown to be confined to the ileo-caecal region. She presents with mild exacerbation of her disease with some diarrhoea and mild abdominal pain. Her weight is stable and her C-reactive protein (CRP) is only slightly elevated. Which of the following statements is correct?

- ☐ **A** Some form of pharmaceutical treatment will be required
- ☐ **B** A 5-ASA compound is better than oral steroids in this situation
- ☐ **C** Budesonide could be used to maintain remission once induced
- ☐ **D** Prednisolone is better than budesonide
- ☐ **E** An elemental diet is an easy to administer alternative to tablets

3.33 A 25-year-old man presents with a history of severe reflux oesophagitis. Which one of the following is the treatment of choice?

- ☐ **A** Antacids only
- ☐ **B** Antireflux surgery
- ☐ **C** H_2-receptor antagonist
- ☐ **D** High-dose proton pump inhibitor (PPI), reducing later
- ☐ **E** Prokinetic therapy

Answers on pages 125–142

3.34 After being treated for bleeding oesophageal varices, an alcoholic patient with ascites is found to have deteriorating renal function. His creatinine is rising each day and his urine output is falling. How would you treat him?

☐ **A** Continuous ambulatory peritoneal dialysis (CAPD)

☐ **B** Dopamine infusion

☐ **C** Intravenous saline

☐ **D** Paracentesis/albumin/glypressin

☐ **E** Spironolactone

3.35 A 26-year-old woman is admitted as an emergency. She has just returned from honeymoon in Goa and her husband reports that she complained of stomach pains and diarrhoea on the return journey a few days ago. She is now intermittently agitated and drowsy and deeply jaundiced. The husband reports that his wife is teetotal. Blood tests are taken and it is noted that the venepuncture site does not stop bleeding after 10 minutes. What is the likely diagnosis?

☐ **A** Paracetamol overdose

☐ **B** Hepatitis A

☐ **C** Hepatitis C

☐ **D** Aspirin overdose

☐ **E** Mushroom poisoning

3.36 A 46-year-old woman is referred by a dermatologist to whom she presented with generalised itching. She was found to have the following biochemical results: bilirubin 34 μmol/l; alanine aminotransferase (ALT) 20 U/l; alkaline phosphatase 380 U/l. Which one of the following is the most likely diagnosis?

☐ **A** Alcoholic cirrhosis

☐ **B** Chronic active hepatitis

☐ **C** Haemochromatosis

☐ **D** Primary biliary cirrhosis

☐ **E** Systemic lupus erythematosus (SLE)

3.37   A 27-year-old intravenous drug user with known HIV disease is noted to
        have abnormal liver function tests and subsequent serological testing
        reveals him to be positive for hepatitis C. He has not injected drugs for 2
        years and remains on a methadone programme. A liver biopsy reveals
        that he has moderate fibrosis but no cirrhosis. Which of the following
        statements is correct?

   □ **A** He is more likely to die of liver disease than AIDS

   □ **B** Hepatitis B vaccination is unlikely to be effective

   □ **C** Combination therapy with ribavirin and interferon is contraindicated

   □ **D** HIV will preclude liver transplantation if disease progresses

   □ **E** Antiretroviral therapy has some activity against the hepatitis C virus

3.38   A 36-year-old alcoholic presents with shock due to bleeding oesophageal
        varices. After resuscitation, which one of the following is the treatment
        of choice?

   □ **A** Sengstaken–Blakemore tube placement

   □ **B** Intravenous glypressin

   □ **C** Oesophageal variceal endoscopic ligation

   □ **D** Intravenous propranolol

   □ **E** Transjugular intrahepatic portosystemic shunt (TIPS)

3.39   A 30-year-old woman with chronic Crohn's disease of the colon is
        planning to have a child. She has required two to three courses of steroid
        each year for the last 5 years. Which one of the following should be
        offered to her?

   □ **A** Azathioprine

   □ **B** Continuous oral prednisolone

   □ **C** Ciclosporin

   □ **D** Infliximab

   □ **E** Methotrexate

3.40 A 42-year-old man is admitted to hospital with abdominal swelling. He
has a history of intravenous drug abuse and heavy alcohol consumption.
On examination he has a grossly distended abdomen with shifting
dullness on percussion. There are scattered spider naevi on his chest and
he is mildly icteric. It is assumed that he has ascites secondary to portal
hypertension and a diagnostic ascitic tap is performed in the medical
assessment ward. Which of the following is true?

- **A** A neutrophil count of > 500 cells/mm^3 indicates spontaneous
  bacterial peritonitis
- **B** If the tap is bloody 60% of cases will be due to hepatocellular
  carcinoma
- **C** Bed rest and sodium restriction 30 mmol/day should be instigated
  immediately
- **D** Placing ascitic fluid into sterile containers for microbiological
  examination will yield an organism in 75% of cases of spontaneous
  bacterial peritonitis
- **E** Serum ascites–albumin gradient (SAAG) is likely to be ⩾ 11 g/l

3.41 A 70-year-old man presents with dysphagia. For 30 years he has
experienced regular episodes of heartburn. An endoscopic biopsy shows
Barrett's oesophagus with high-grade dysplasia. Which one of the
following would you use in the first instance to treat this patient?

- **A** Antireflux surgery
- **B** Laser ablation
- **C** Oesophagectomy
- **D** Proton pump inhibitor (PPI) treatment with repeat endoscopy in 3 to 6
  months
- **E** Proton pump inhibitor alone

3.42 **A 46-year-old woman presents with rectal bleeding. She reports that she has had difficult defecation for some years and has had to strain to pass her stools, which are hard. The blood she has observed coats or follows her stool, rather than being mixed with it. Sigmoidoscopy reveals a raised ulcerated lesion on the anterior wall of the lower rectum. Which one of the following is the most likely diagnosis?**

☐ **A** Crohn's disease

☐ **B** Haemorrhoids

☐ **C** Lymphogranuloma venereum (LGV)

☐ **D** Rectal carcinoma

☐ **E** Solitary rectal ulcer

3.43 **A 70-year-old Egyptian man with a long history of chronic obstructive pulmonary disease (COPD) presents with a 6-month history of diarrhoea and rectal bleeding. Sigmoidoscopy reveals polypoid lesions lining the mucosa of the rectum and at barium enema the left colon is reported as looking 'like bubble wrap'. What is the most likely diagnosis?**

☐ **A** Antibiotic diarrhoea

☐ **B** Familial adenomatous polyposis

☐ **C** Pneumatosis coli

☐ **D** Schistosomiasis

☐ **E** Villous rectal cancer

3.44 **A 36-year-old man presents with painless rectal bleeding. He is a gay man and has had several sexual relationships in the months before his symptoms. There are no signs on physical examination except on sigmoidoscopy, which shows a florid proctitis. Biopsies show inclusion bodies in the mucosa. Which one of the following is the correct diagnosis?**

☐ **A** Cytomegalovirus (CMV) proctitis

☐ **B** Herpes

☐ **C** Lymphogranuloma venereum (LGV)

☐ **D** Solitary rectal ulcer

☐ **E** Syphilis

Answers on pages 125–142

3.45   A 20-year-old man presents with massive haematemesis. He drinks little
        alcohol and does not inject drugs. His past medical history is
        unremarkable except for a prolonged stay on the Special Care Baby Unit
        (SCBU) after being born prematurely. His spleen is palpable, but he has
        no stigmata of chronic liver disease. Which one of the following is the
        underlying diagnosis?

    □ **A** Cirrhosis secondary to hepatitis C

    □ **B** Cryptogenic cirrhosis

    □ **C** Lymphoma

    □ **D** Portal vein thrombosis

    □ **E** Primary biliary cirrhosis

3.46   A 60-year-old Welsh sheep farmer is admitted for routine hip
        replacement surgery. On examination he is noted to have hepatomegaly.
        Ultrasonography reveals multiple cystic lesions with echogenic areas
        within the cysts. Which one of the following is the most likely diagnosis?

    □ **A** Haemangioma

    □ **B** Hydatid disease

    □ **C** Necrotic metastases

    □ **D** Polycystic disease

    □ **E** Simple hepatic cysts

3.47   **Which of the following is true regarding cholecystokinin?**

    □ A In excess, it precipitates gallstones

    □ B It causes delayed gastric emptying through its action as a smooth
                muscle relaxant

    □ C It is found in higher concentrations following cholecystectomy

    □ D It releases the ileal brake

    □ E It stimulates pancreatic exocrine secretion

3.48 One week after a colectomy with ileostomy for ulcerative colitis, a 26-year-old woman begins to experience stomal diarrhoea. The pain around her stoma had started to settle, but increased again. Investigations show her C-reactive protein (CRP) level to have risen and her albumin level to have fallen. Which one of the following is the cause of her problem?

☐ **A** Antibiotic diarrhoea

☐ **B** Bile salt diarrhoea

☐ **C** Functional diarrhoea due to her disquiet about her stoma

☐ **D** *Clostridium difficile* infection

☐ **E** Peristomal abscess

3.49 A 24-year-old man with severe Crohn's disease is looking likely to require his third small bowel resection in 5 years. While considering the consequences of his surgery, which of the following is true?

☐ **A** The length of resected bowel must be measured as it determines likely outcome

☐ **B** If he has a jejuno-colic anastomosis he is likely to require long-term parenteral nutrition

☐ **C** Hypomagnesaemia may become a problem

☐ **D** If he has a jejunostomy he must be encouraged to drink large volumes of water

☐ **E** He will be at increased risk of renal calculi

3.50 After eating a very large Sunday lunch, a 42-year-old man vomits several times before experiencing severe chest pain. On presentation to the Emergency Department, he is shocked. His electrocardiogram (ECG) is normal, but his chest X-ray (CXR) shows some shadowing in the left lower zone. Which one of the following is the diagnosis?

☐ **A** Boerhaave's syndrome

☐ **B** Gastritis

☐ **C** Mallory–Weiss tear

☐ **D** Myocardial infarction

☐ **E** Oesophagitis

Answers on pages 125–142

Nephrology

Best of Five

Questions

NEPHROLOGY: 'BEST OF FIVE' QUESTIONS

For each of the questions select the ONE most appropriate answer from the options provided.

4.1   Which of the following is true about the loop of Henle?

☐ **A** Fluid entering the distal tubule is hypo-osmolar

☐ **B** ANP causes an increase in urinary water excretion by its action on the descending limb

☐ **C** Aquaporin channels are concentrated in the ascending limb

☐ **D** Amiloride blocks Na-Cl co-transporters in the distal tubule

☐ **E** The medullary interstitium is iso-osmotic at every depth

4.2   A 35-year-old woman attends her GP surgery complaining of a 3-month history of weight loss and fatigue. Direct questioning reveals additional symptoms of small joint arthralgia, pleuritic chest pain and hair loss. Investigations reveal a serum creatinine of 210 µmol/l, haemoglobin (Hb) 10.1 g/dl, erythrocyte sedimentation rate (ESR) 90 mm/h and urinalysis: protein +++, blood +. She is referred to renal clinic. Which will be the most likely histological finding on renal biopsy?

☐ **A** Diffuse proliferative glomerulonephritis

☐ **B** Pauci-immune focal necrotising glomerulonephritis with crescent formation

☐ **C** Interstitial nephritis

☐ **D** Cholesterol crystals

☐ **E** Congo red staining

4.3 A 52-year-old man is seen in the Out-patients' Department with a serum creatinine of 210 µmol/l. Urinalysis reveals protein + blood –. He has been a smoker of 10 per day for 30 years. On examination he has a blood pressure of 180/90 mmHg. Otherwise examination is unremarkable except for absent foot pulses. Routine electrocardiogram (ECG) reveals left bundle branch block. Renal ultrasound is reported as showing a right kidney with bipolar length 10.7 cm, normal cortical depth; left kidney 8.1 cm with cortical thinning. No hydronephrosis. What is the next investigation of choice?

- ☐ **A** Renal angiogram
- ☐ **B** Biopsy of left kidney
- ☐ **C** Biopsy of right kidney
- ☐ **D** MRA of renal arteries
- ☐ **E** Intravenous pyelogram (IVP)

4.4 A 37-year-old woman is referred to a renal clinic with a 3-week history of dependent oedema. The GP has found her to have proteinuria, quantified at 5.8 g per 24 h. Serum creatinine is normal. Which of the following clinical findings is likely to be aetiologically useful?

- ☐ **A** Blood pressure (BP) 200/110 mmHg
- ☐ **B** Needle track marks
- ☐ **C** Hot swollen unilateral tender calf
- ☐ **D** Unilateral ptosis
- ☐ **E** Facial oedema

4.5 Which of the following is true of proximal renal tubular acidosis (type II)?

- ☐ **A** It is characterised by severe hypokalaemia
- ☐ **B** Nephrocalcinosis is rare
- ☐ **C** The acidosis is easily correctible by small doses of bicarbonate
- ☐ **D** It is a recognised complication of amiodarone therapy
- ☐ **E** It is caused by an inability of the tubular cells to secrete enough H^+ ions

4.6 A 27-year-old man is admitted to hospital after visiting his GP complaining of fatigue. Screening blood tests revealed haemoglobin (Hb) 8.3 g/dl, serum creatinine 356 μmol/l. Urinalysis shows a trace of protein. He has never had a blood test before. Which of the following statements are correct about the chronicity of his condition?

- ☐ **A** Absence of significant proteinuria suggests acute renal failure
- ☐ **B** Anaemia is indicative of chronic renal disease
- ☐ **C** If the renal ultrasound shows large kidneys the condition may be chronic
- ☐ **D** Raised phosphate levels indicate chronic renal disease
- ☐ **E** If the ultrasound shows bright kidneys the condition is probably acute

4.7 A 54-year-old woman is admitted with a 3-week history of increasing breathlessness and haemoptysis. On admission she has $p(O_2)$ 8.6 kPa, $p(CO_2)$ 4.5 kPa, potassium 6.1 mmol/l, creatinine 478 μmol/l. She is oliguric. Chest X-ray shows patchy opacification throughout both lung fields. Antineutrophil cytoplasmic antibody (ANCA) was positive at a dilution of 1:320, with a pattern of diffuse cytoplasmic staining. An urgent renal biopsy is performed, which shows crescentic glomerulonephritis with linear immunofluorescence along the basement membrane. What investigation is now most likely to be diagnostic?

- ☐ **A** ASO titres
- ☐ **B** Anti-GBM assay
- ☐ **C** Anti-dsDNA titres
- ☐ **D** ELISA for MPO antibodies
- ☐ **E** Trans-oesophageal echocardiogram

4.8   A 41-year-old man with chronic renal failure due to diabetes mellitus is
under regular follow-up in the renal clinic. His current medication
consists of actrapid, insulatard, lisinopril, bisoprolol, erythropoietin beta,
aspirin, and sevelamer. His latest blood results show serum creatinine
436 µmol/l, corrected calcium 2.12 mmol/l, phosphate 1.52 mmol/l,
parathyroid hormone (PTH) 34 pmol/l (normal range 1–5). Which of the
following treatments is advisable?

☐ **A** Parathyroidectomy

☐ **B** Calcichew after meals plus alfacalcidol

☐ **C** Calcichew before meals plus risedronate

☐ **D** Risedronate alone

☐ **E** Alfacalcidol alone

4.9   A 55-year-old man with hypertension was treated by his GP with
ramipril. Ten days later his serum creatinine had risen from a baseline of
100 µmol/l to a level of 183. A presumptive diagnosis of renal artery
disease was made, and the serum creatinine fell after the ramipril was
discontinued. Which of the following is the best explanation for his acute
renal failure?

☐ **A** Ramipril can cause interstitial nephritis in susceptible people

☐ **B** Ramipril reduces the conversion of angiotensin I to angiotensin II, so
causing hypotension and consequent acute renal failure

☐ **C** Ramipril blocks the action of aldosterone on the renal tubules,
resulting in sodium wasting and consequent reduction in circulating
volume

☐ **D** Ramipril causes a preferential dilatation of the efferent glomerular
arteriole resulting in a critical fall in glomerular filtration pressure

☐ **E** Ramipril desensitises the juxtaglomerular apparatus to changes in renal
perfusion, which blunts the angiotensin response to hypotension

4.10 A 27-year-old woman is admitted to hospital 3 weeks after the spontaneous vaginal delivery of her second child. Both pregnancies have been entirely uneventful. In particular, there is no history of pre-eclampsia. She has had no prodromal illness, and is on no regular medication. One week ago, she visited her GP complaining of severe headaches. Her blood pressure (BP) at that time was 150/100 mmHg. Two days later, she began vomiting. Two days later again, she became confused and oliguric. On examination she has a Glasgow Coma Scale (GCS) rating of 10. She is apyrexial, P90, BP 240/130 mmHg. She has no bruising or petechiae. Chest is clear. Heart sounds normal. Abdomen reveals a firm mass arising from the pelvis approximately 4 cm above the symphysis pubis. She has a brownish vaginal discharge. Fundoscopy reveals grade III hypertensive changes. Blood tests are as follows: haemoglobin (Hb) 6.3 g/dl; platelets 37×10^3/mm³; clotting screen normal; creatinine 487 µmol/l. What is the most likely diagnosis?

☐ **A** Disseminated intravascular coagulation (DIC)

☐ **B** Thrombotic thrombocytopenic purpura (TTP)

☐ **C** Haemolytic uraemic syndrome (HUS)

☐ **D** Toxic shock syndrome

☐ **E** Delayed-onset pre-eclampsia

4.11 Which of the following causes of end-stage renal failure is most likely to exhibit clinically significant recurrence in a renal transplant?

☐ **A** Membranous glomerulonephritis

☐ **B** Systemic lupus erythematosus (SLE)

☐ **C** Diabetic nephropathy

☐ **D** IgA nephropathy

☐ **E** Focal segmental glomerulosclerosis

4.12 **A 62-year-old White woman is being investigated for hypertension and chronic renal failure (serum creatinine 210 µmol/l). Intravenous pyelogram (IVP) shows irregular-shaped kidneys with calyceal blunting. Which of the following elements from her history and examination is likely to be aetiologically relevant?**

☐ **A** Falciparum malaria 3 years ago.

☐ **B** A family history of beta thalassaemia

☐ **C** Chronic lumbar spine pain

☐ **D** Occupational exposure to hydrocarbons

☐ **E** Liquorice addiction

4.13 **Which of the following is a strong indication for the selection of haemodialysis over peritoneal dialysis when determining long-term dialysis modality?**

☐ **A** Chronic obstructive pulmonary disease

☐ **B** Patient is visually impaired

☐ **C** Diabetes mellitus

☐ **D** Cardiovascular disease

☐ **E** Patient with difficulty adhering to fluid restriction

4.14 **A comatose 18-year-old girl has acute renal failure 2 days after taking a multiple drug overdose. For the removal of which drug is haemodialysis most likely to be effective?**

☐ **A** Amiodarone

☐ **B** Digoxin

☐ **C** Lithium

☐ **D** Paraquat

☐ **E** Phenytoin

Answers on pages 145–160

4.15 **In a 45-year-old man with acute renal failure, which one of the following is most likely to be correct?**

☐ **A** Hyaline casts on urinalysis suggest a glomerulonephritis

☐ **B** In oliguria, dopamine should be used to promote a diuresis

☐ **C** Low plasma sodium reflects salt-wasting in the renal tubule

☐ **D** Non-oliguria carries a better prognosis for long-term renal function than oliguria

☐ **E** Obstruction is excluded by polyuria

4.16 **In which one of the following circumstances is renal excretion of water most likely to be increased?**

☐ **A** Chronic renal failure

☐ **B** Early phase of acute tubular necrosis

☐ **C** Hyperkalaemia

☐ **D** Hypokalaemia

☐ **E** Secondary hyperaldosteronism

4.17 **In a woman who is 36 weeks' pregnant, which one of the following results is a cause for concern?**

☐ **A** Creatinine 85 μmol/l

☐ **B** Glomerular filtration rate (GFR) 149 ml/min

☐ **C** Magnesium 0.4 mmol/l

☐ **D** Urate 0.7 mmol/l

☐ **E** Urea 1 mmol/l

4.18 **In a normal-functioning kidney, which one of the following is most likely to increase urinary sodium excretion?**

☐ **A** Decrease in glomerular filtration rate (GFR) of 10%

☐ **B** Fall in renal arterial pressure of 15 mmHg

☐ **C** Increase in plasma protein concentration

☐ **D** Increase in renal sympathetic nervous activity

☐ **E** Increase in venous volume

4.19 **A healthy individual has arterial blood gases measured at 10 000 feet. The arterial $p_a(CO_2)$ is low. Which one of the following best represents the renal response to this fall in $p_a(CO_2)$?**

☐ **A** Compensation by a rise in pH

☐ **B** Compensation predominantly occurring at the proximal tubule

☐ **C** Full correction of blood gas measurement of carbon dioxide

☐ **D** The renal response leads to a rise in plasma bicarbonate

☐ **E** The renal response leads to volume expansion

4.20 **In a healthy individual which one of the following is an accurate statement regarding renin?**

☐ **A** Decreased renin release increases thirst

☐ **B** Decreased renin release leads indirectly to vasoconstriction

☐ **C** Renal cortical ischaemia does not lead to increased renin release

☐ **D** Renin release decreases in response to sodium depletion

☐ **E** Renal sympathetic nervous stimulation causes increased renin release

4.21 **A 40-year-old man is found to be uraemic. Which one of the following facts from the history is most suggestive of a diagnosis of retroperitoneal fibrosis?**

☐ **A** He had childhood haematuria

☐ **B** He previously worked in an iron foundry

☐ **C** He takes atenolol for hypertension

☐ **D** He takes paracetamol for fibrositis

☐ **E** Three of his children had haemolytic disease of the newborn

4.22 **Which one of the following diagnoses is most likely to be correctly made utilising the renal imaging investigations given?**

☐ **A** Dehydration by good quality intravenous urograms

☐ **B** Normal renal histology by 13 cm kidneys on ultrasound

☐ **C** Reflux nephropathy by coarse kidney scarring on intravenous urograms

☐ **D** Renal obstruction by static radionuclide scanning

☐ **E** Retroperitoneal fibrosis by medial ureteric displacement on intravenous urograms

Answers on pages 145–160

4.23 **A 33-year-old woman presents with nephrotic syndrome and membranous glomerulonephritis is suspected. Which one of the following is most likely to support this diagnosis?**

☐ **A** End-stage renal failure occurring within 6 months of presentation

☐ **B** Highly selective proteinuria

☐ **C** IgM deposits within the basement membrane

☐ **D** Previous presentation with nephritic syndrome

☐ **E** Gold therapy for rheumatoid arthritis

4.24 **Which one of the following statements is the most accurate concerning IgA nephropathy?**

☐ **A** Glomerular crescents may occur during episodes of macroscopic haematuria

☐ **B** It is an uncommon form of glomerulonephritis

☐ **C** Loin pain may occur due to bleeding from peripheral renal arteries

☐ **D** Most patients affected will require dialysis treatment

☐ **E** The degree of proteinuria does not relate to prognosis

4.25 **A 64-year-old man with renal failure develops acute loin pain and haematuria. Doppler ultrasound confirms he has a renal vein thrombosis. Which one of the following is the most likely underlying disease?**

☐ **A** Chronic pyelonephritis

☐ **B** IgA glomerulonephritis

☐ **C** Interstitial nephritis

☐ **D** Reflux nephropathy

☐ **E** Renal amyloidosis

4.26 **Patients with which one of the following inherited diseases are most likely to have a renal tubular defect?**

☐ **A** Childhood polycystic kidney disease

☐ **B** Cystinosis

☐ **C** Noonan's syndrome

☐ **D** Vesico-ureteric reflux

☐ **E** von Hippel–Lindau syndrome

4.27 **A 55-year-old woman presents with renal failure. Which one of the following features is most consistent with a diagnosis of vesico-ureteric reflux?**

- ☐ **A** History of childhood enuresis
- ☐ **B** Normal DMSA (dimercaptosuccinic acid) scan
- ☐ **C** Normal micturating cystourethrography
- ☐ **D** Positive antineutrophil cytoplasmic antibody (ANCA)
- ☐ **E** Presentation with acute renal failure

4.28 **In an Asian man with active tuberculosis of the urinary tract, which one of the following is most likely to occur?**

- ☐ **A** Microscopic haematuria
- ☐ **B** Night sweats
- ☐ **C** Normal chest X-ray
- ☐ **D** Persistent pyuria
- ☐ **E** Raised serum angiotensin-converting enzyme (ACE) levels

4.29 **In a patient who is approaching end-stage renal failure, which one of the following drugs is the safest to use?**

- ☐ **A** Ibuprofen
- ☐ **B** Lisinopril
- ☐ **C** Mesalazine
- ☐ **D** Omeprazole
- ☐ **E** Oxytetracycline

4.30 **Which one of the following is true with regard to cholesterol embolisation?**

- ☐ **A** It is a rare cause of renal damage
- ☐ **B** It is best diagnosed by arteriography
- ☐ **C** It is often associated with blue mottling of the hands
- ☐ **D** It is usually manifest by loin pain and frank haematuria
- ☐ **E** It is often associated with eosinophilia

Answers on pages 145–160

4.31 **Which one of the following is true of hepatitis C infection with regard to the kidney?**

☐ **A** Membranous glomerulonephritis is typical

☐ **B** Pulsed methylprednisolone may be used in treatment

☐ **C** Renal remission is rare

☐ **D** The disease is mediated by cold agglutinins

☐ **E** There is direct viral infection of the glomerular endothelium

4.32 **Which one of the following is typical of a renal biopsy in a patient with diabetic nephropathy?**

☐ **A** Diffuse glomerular capillary thickening and basement membrane spikes

☐ **B** Green birefringence on staining with Congo red

☐ **C** Intracapillary hyaline thrombi

☐ **D** Mesangial hypercellularity and fibrinoid necrosis

☐ **E** Mesangial widening, basement membrane thickening and capillary obliteration

4.33 **Which one of the following is characteristic of vitamin D-resistant rickets?**

☐ **A** Elevated 1,25-dihydroxycholecalciferol

☐ **B** Expression confined to males

☐ **C** Glycosuria

☐ **D** Impaired phosphate excretion

☐ **E** Normal parathyroid hormone levels

4.34 **Which one of the following is true of the complications of renal transplantation?**

☐ **A** Cytomegalovirus (CMV) matching of donor and recipient is essential

☐ **B** Gastric ulceration is partly attributable to increased rate of *Helicobacter pylori* carriage

☐ **C** *Pneumocystis* infection typically occurs at around 1 year posttransplant

☐ **D** Reverse barrier nursing for 10 days after surgery is mandatory

☐ **E** The major cause of mortality is malignancy

4.35 **Which one of the following is true for most patients with moderate chronic renal impairment?**

☐ **A** Alcohol is contraindicated

☐ **B** Dairy products are a useful source of calcium

☐ **C** Fluid intake should be 2–3 litres per day

☐ **D** The diet should be high in cholesterol

☐ **E** Very low protein diet is beneficial

4.36 **Which one of the following is true of renal involvement in HIV infection?**

☐ **A** Antiviral therapy is of little benefit in HIV-associated nephropathy

☐ **B** HIV-associated nephropathy is indistinguishable histologically from focal segmental glomerulosclerosis

☐ **C** HIV-associated nephropathy typically presents with nephrotic-range proteinuria

☐ **D** Hypernatraemia is common in HIV infection

☐ **E** Renal involvement is common in AIDS

4.37 **Which one of the following is therapeutically useful in cystinuria?**

☐ **A** Allopurinol

☐ **B** Cysteamine

☐ **C** Desferrioxamine

☐ **D** Penicillamine

☐ **E** Potassium citrate

4.38 **Which of the following is useful in the treatment of renal stone disease?**

☐ **A** Spironolactone

☐ **B** Colestyramine

☐ **C** Ibuprofen

☐ **D** Captopril

☐ **E** Pantoprazole

Answers on pages 145–160

4.39 A 24-year-old known epileptic is admitted to the Emergency Department in status epilepticus. He is treated with intravenous phenytoin. Some 48 hours later he is found to have acute renal failure. Blood results are as follows: potassium 7.1 mmol/l, creatinine 782 µmol/l, corrected calcium 1.9 mmol/l, phosphate 3.1 mmol/l. What simple procedure would be most useful diagnostically?

- ☐ **A** BM stix
- ☐ **B** Electrocardiogram
- ☐ **C** Fundoscopy
- ☐ **D** Plain abdominal X-ray
- ☐ **E** Dipstick urinalysis and microscopy

4.40 Which one of the following is not typically associated with reduced serum complement activity?

- ☐ **A** Acute poststreptococcal nephritis
- ☐ **B** Antiglomerular basement membrane disease
- ☐ **C** Essential mixed cryoglobulinaemia
- ☐ **D** Lupus nephritis
- ☐ **E** Type II mesangiocapillary glomerulonephritis

4.41 Which one of the following examination findings in a patient with renal disease is likely to be helpful in determining the aetiology of the condition described?

- ☐ **A** Adenoma sebaceum in a patient with microscopic haematuria
- ☐ **B** Grade 2 hypertensive retinopathy in a patient presenting with creatinine of 647 µmol/l
- ☐ **C** Corneal arcus in a patient with proteinuria of 7 g/24 h
- ☐ **D** Partial lipodystrophy in a patient with a creatinine of 150 µmol/l and normal urinary sediment
- ☐ **E** Truncal obesity, thin skin and striae in a patient with a creatinine of 270 µmol/l and proteinuria of 1.5 g/24 h

4.42 **Which one of the following features would make a diagnosis of poststreptococcal glomerulonephritis unlikely?**

☐ **A** Infection 2 weeks ago with α-haemolytic *Streptococcus*

☐ **B** Patient is a 7-year-old girl

☐ **C** Proteinuria of 1.1 g/24 h

☐ **D** No elevation of antistreptolysin titre

☐ **E** No impairment of renal function at presentation

4.43 **Which one of the following is true with regard to blood pressure and pregnancy?**

☐ **A** Eclampsia can occur without previous hypertension

☐ **B** It is important to use Korotkoff phase V for blood pressure measurement

☐ **C** The accepted threshold for physiological proteinuria is 0.8 g/24 h

☐ **D** The physiological fall in blood pressure is due to reduced cardiac work

☐ **E** The risk of pre-eclampsia increases with each subsequent pregnancy

4.44 **Which one of the following is true with regard to proteinuria?**

☐ **A** Urinary protein excretion of 3 g/l, in conjunction with microscopic haematuria, may be attributable to strenuous exercise

☐ **B** In orthostatic proteinuria, the proteinuria is only present in recumbency

☐ **C** Membranous glomerulonephritis is a major cause of the nephrotic syndrome in young adults

☐ **D** Microalbuminuria is diagnosed by Albustix testing

☐ **E** Pathological proteinuria is pathognomonic of glomerular pathology

Answers on pages 145–160

4.45 **Which one of the following patients is least likely to develop clinically evident diabetic nephropathy within the next year?**

- [ ] **A** A 43-year-old man who has had type 1 diabetes mellitus (DM) for 11 years, and who has early retinopathy
- [ ] **B** A 50-year-old woman with no past medical history, found on routine testing to have glycosuria +++
- [ ] **C** A 60-year-old man who developed type 1 DM 43 years ago
- [ ] **D** A White subject 17 years after development of type 2 DM
- [ ] **E** A Japanese subject 17 years after development of type 2 DM

4.46 **In a healthy man on a normal diet, which of the following is true?**

- [ ] **A** The minimum required water intake is approximately 0.8 litres per day
- [ ] **B** The net insensible water loss is approximately 0.2 litres per day
- [ ] **C** The obligated urine volume is approximately 1.3 litres per day
- [ ] **D** Water intake of 10 litres in one day would not result in hyponatraemia
- [ ] **E** Water loss in stools is approximately 0.5 litres per day

4.47 **Which one of the following is the most important cause of death among UK patients with end-stage renal failure (ESRF)?**

- [ ] **A** Cardiac/vascular
- [ ] **B** Complications of transplantation
- [ ] **C** Infection
- [ ] **D** Malignancy
- [ ] **E** Voluntary withdrawal of dialysis/suicide

4.48 **Which one of the following statements concerning haematuria is true?**

- [ ] **A** A high proportion of distorted red cells suggests a tubular origin
- [ ] **B** Family history is unlikely to be relevant
- [ ] **C** Haematuria becomes visible at a concentration of approximately 20 ml blood per litre of urine
- [ ] **D** Microscopic haematuria is a normal finding in warfarinised patients
- [ ] **E** 1 g per day of proteinuria would be expected with haematuria due to a bladder malignancy

4.49 **Which one of the following is likely to be therapeutically useful in a patient suffering from hepatorenal syndrome?**

☐ **A** Angiotensin-converting enzyme (ACE) inhibition

☐ **B** Combined liver and kidney transplantation

☐ **C** Continuous veno-venous haemofiltration

☐ **D** Correction of hyponatraemia with normal saline infusion

☐ **E** Volume expansion with colloid

4.50 **In the investigation of a neonate with renal cysts, which one of the following is most likely to allow differentiation between autosomal recessive and autosomal dominant polycystic disease?**

☐ **A** Intravenous pyelogram (IVP) of patient

☐ **B** Liver ultrasonography of patient

☐ **C** Renal biopsy of patient

☐ **D** Renal ultrasonography of patient

☐ **E** Renal ultrasonography of teenage parents

ANSWERS

Clinical Pharmacology

CLINICAL PHARMACOLOGY: 'BEST OF FIVE' ANSWERS

1.1   B: Diclofenac

There is a number of potential causes of impaired renal function in this lady, not least of which her diabetes itself, perhaps unmasked by an intercurrent infection. However, drugs should always be considered as potential aetiologies. The distinction needs to be made between those drugs that cause toxicity in the setting of renal failure (perhaps because they are entirely renally excreted) and those drugs that are directly nephrotoxic. This question is asking about the latter rather than the former. Metformin is handled almost exclusively by the kidneys and is contraindicated in the presence of even mild renal impairment because of the risk of lactic acidosis. Digoxin and trimethoprim similarly can produce toxicity in the setting of renal dysfunction. On the other hand there are other drugs that can be directly nephrotoxic including non-steroidal anti-inflammatory drugs (NSAIDs) and aminoglycosides.

1.2   B: Co-amoxiclav

Prescribing for patients with porphyria needs great care and advice should always be sought for the latest information. Many drugs can induce acute porphyric crises. The British National Formulary gives a list of drugs known to be, or believed to be, unsafe in porphyria. This list includes amphetamines, antidepressants (although fluoxetine is felt to be safe), barbiturates, progestogens and oestrogens as well as drugs like statins and sulphonyl ureas. Carbamazepine and erythromycin should also be avoided in acute porphyria. Treatment of serious or life-threatening conditions in these patients should however not be withheld in the absence of an alternative and monitoring of urinary porphobilinogen excretion may be undertaken. There are drugs that are considered to be safe in porphyria and this includes the penicillins (eg: co-amoxiclav and flucloxacillin), opiates and β-blockers.

1.3   D: Nifedipine

This is a question about a specific adverse drug reaction that may be associated with a number of drugs. As such this question can only be approached by knowledge of those drugs that commonly cause this particular problem. In this case nifedipine is the culprit. Although phenytoin is associated with gum hypertrophy, carbamazepine is not. Ciclosporin is another drug that can cause gingival hypertrophy.

1.4   D: Erythromycin

Warfarin is a commonly used drug with a relatively narrow therapeutic index and is also prone to a number of potentially significant drug interactions. Warfarin is predominantly metabolised by the cytochrome P450 isoenzyme CYP2C9 and this is inhibited by erythromycin – an example of a pharmacokinetic drug–drug interaction. If such treatment is required then the patient will need close pharmacodynamic monitoring (through measurement of the international normalised ratio) during and following therapy. The anticoagulant effect of warfarin may be enhanced by intensive broad-spectrum antimicrobial therapy (such as with penicillins and cephalosporins) by reducing the intestinal flora that produce vitamin K. This however is an example of a pharmacodynamic interaction. Studies have failed to show any significant interaction with trimethoprim.

1.5   A: Abacavir

Life-threatening hypersensitivity reactions to abacavir are well reported and occur in about 6% of patients. These reactions are characterised by a wide range of symptoms, typically fever or rash, as well as gastrointestinal disturbance or full-blown anaphylaxis. The symptoms usually appear within the first 6 weeks of treatment, but they may occur at any time. The drug should be stopped immediately and not restarted as rechallenge can result in a more severe reaction that can be fatal.

1.6   C: Amiodarone has β-adrenoceptor blocking activity

Amiodarone is a broad-spectrum anti-arrhythmic drug used in a variety of supra-ventricular and ventricular arrhythmias, particularly when other drugs are ineffective or are contraindicated. Amiodarone prolongs the effective refractory period of myocardial cells, thereby prolonging the action potential (and QT interval) – a class III agent according to the Vaughan–Williams classification of anti-arrhythmic drugs. Amiodarone also specifically prolongs the effective refractory period within the arteriovenous (AV) node and anomalous pathways, as well as acting as a non-competitive inhibitor at β-adrenoceptors. The pharmacokinetics of amiodarone are notable because of its very long half-life and its enormous apparent volume of distribution. It takes many weeks (or even months) to achieve steady-state plasma concentrations. Most people taking amiodarone therapy develop corneal microdeposits, which are typically reversible on the cessation of therapy. Less commonly, pulmonary fibrosis (and hepatitis) occur, and sometimes this can develop rapidly even during short-term use of the drug.

1.7   A: Amlodipine

Gynaecomastia can be caused by a wide range of drugs, predictably including those drugs that are either oestrogen-like or anti-androgen. In this patient the culprit drug is a calcium channel blocker as gynaecomastia is not well recognised or reported in any of the others listed. Spironolactone certainly causes gynaecomastia but not furosemide. Other causes are: stilboestrol, cyproterone, goserelin, steroids, cimetidine, omeprazole, sodium valproate, digoxin, amiodarone and the dopamine receptor antagonists.

1.8   E: Thrombocytopenia

The phenomenon of heparin-induced thrombocytopenia is well recognised and immune mediated. It typically does not develop until at least 6 days treatment has been given, and hence regular platelet counts are recommended for patients receiving heparin for longer than 5 days. *Hyper*kalaemia is also a potential problem of this length of heparin treatment through inhibition of aldosterone secretion, particularly in those patients prone to hyperkalaemia anyway (those with renal failure or those taking potassium-sparing diuretics). Osteoporosis certainly is an adverse effect associated with all heparin therapy (including low-molecular-weight heparin) but only after prolonged use, and that would not be encountered in the circumstances described here.

1.9   B: Chlorpromazine

The biochemistry is consistent with cholestasis. Ascertaining that the abnormalities are drug related is difficult and is usually a diagnosis of exclusion once other investigations looking for other aetiologies have been completed (ultrasound scan, hepatitis serology etc). Drugs causing cholestasis include chlorpromazine, erythromycin, co-amoxiclav, nitrofurantoin, cimetidine and chlorpropamide. A hepatitic picture is more commonly seen with drugs such as amiodarone, isoniazid and methyldopa. The glitazones (thiazolidinediones) can also cause hepatitis. Metformin does not typically perturb liver function, but hepatitis has been reported.

1.10   C: Renal and thyroid function should be monitored at least once a year

Lithium salts have a narrow therapeutic index and therefore therapeutic drug monitoring is an essential part of management in all patients. Doses are adjusted to achieve serum lithium concentrations of between 0.4 and 1.0 mmol/l on samples taken 12 hours after the preceding dose – levels greater than 2.0 mmol/l would be associated with severe toxicity and require emergency management. Lithium toxicity is made worse by anything that leads to sodium depletion, including vomiting, adrenocortical insufficiency, and commonly diuretic therapy. Renal and thyroid function should be monitored every 6 to 12 months. Weight gain can be a problem during treatment, with or without oedema. The long-term use of lithium has been associated with, not only thyroid dysfunction, but also cognitive and memory impairment. Hence this treatment should not be undertaken lightly without specialist supervision.

1.11   A: Aspirin

As more women survive significant cardiovascular disease, and become pregnant later in life, this is an increasingly common clinical problem. A number of factors aside from the inherent toxicity of the drug play a part. The dose ingested is very important, as are the bioavailability of the drug and the clearance of the drug in the neonate. Heparin (both unfractionated and low-molecular-weight heparins) and warfarin will cross into breast milk, but at normal therapeutic doses taken by the mother, the amount reaching the neonate will be too small to achieve any significant clinical effect (ie anticoagulation). Clopidogrel is best avoided in breast-feeding, but aspirin's effects are well characterised and should be absolutely contraindicated in breast-feeding. Aspirin can cause neonatal bleeding as well as Reye's syndrome. Many other commonly used drugs such as non-steroidal anti-inflammatory drugs (NSAIDs), carbamazepine, penicillins, erythromycin and thyroxine are all relatively safe in breast-feeding.

1.12   A: Carbamazepine

Stevens–Johnson Syndrome (SJS) is an immune-complex-mediated hypersensitivity syndrome that is a severe form of erythema multiforme. SJS typically involves the skin and the mucous membranes. There may be a minor presentation or more significant involvement of oral, nasal, eye, vaginal, urethral, gastrointestinal, and lower respiratory tract mucous membranes. Gastrointestinal and respiratory involvement may progress to necrosis with the potential for severe morbidity. SJS can be fatal. Drugs, infections and malignancy are the major aetiological categories, although a significant proportion remains idiopathic. Almost any drug can potentially cause SJS although the drugs most commonly implicated are the anticonvulsants, penicillin, sulphur-containing antibiotics and anti-inflammatories.

1.13   A: Amitriptyline

The clinical picture is consistent with a tricyclic antidepressant overdose. This class of drugs presents with a varied clinical picture typically with anti-cholinergic features predominating – clinical features such as dry mouth, dilated pupils and urinary retention are relatively common. Altered conscious level, hyperthermia, hypotension, convulsions and arrhythmias are also seen. Treatment is essentially supportive and expectant dealing with problems as they arise: maintenance of a clear airway, intravenous benzodiazepines for seizures and the use of sodium bicarbonate in the presence of electrocardiogram (ECG) abnormalities, including those with QRS prolongation.

1.14   D: Ciprofloxacin and theophylline

Drug interactions are common questions. Lots of drugs interact, either in terms of pharmacokinetics or pharmacodynamics and sometimes this is used to therapeutic advantage. The clinically significant drug interactions are predominantly those that affect drugs with a relatively narrow therapeutic index: so drugs like warfarin, ciclosporin, phenytoin, theophyllines and sulphonyl ureas are prime targets. The interactions can lead to therapeutic failure or, more problematically, toxicity. Ciprofloxacin inhibits the capacity of the liver to metabolise theophylline and therefore high concentrations may result in toxicity. The other drugs listed are commonly given in combination and are not associated with clinically significant problems. There is probably no pharmacological sense behind giving codeine and tramadol at the same time, although it is commonly seen on prescriptions.

1.15   B: Commission on Human Medicines (CHM)

The Medicines Control Agency (MCA) and Medical Devices Agency (MDA) became a single agency to form the Medicines and Healthcare Products Regulatory Agency (MHRA), the government body charged with the responsibility for making sure that medicines and medical devices are acceptably safe, through drug licensing (marketing authorisations) and pharmacovigilance (essentially monitoring of drug safety). These responsibilities are devolved to an independent committee, the Commission on Human Medicines (formerly the Committee on Safety of Medicines). This Commission oversees the Yellow Card Adverse Drug Reaction reporting scheme for instance. NICE are most concerned with the efficacy, clinical utility and cost-effectiveness of drugs in a publicly funded health system like the NHS, and the NPSA has a number of remits, all within the wider scope of patient safety.

1.16   B: Insulin resistance

Protease inhibitors inhibit the viral aspartyl protease. They have largely been used in combination with two nucleoside analogues: such regimens have been shown to retard disease progression and decrease mortality. Protease inhibitors inhibit the cytochrome P450 enzymes and can therefore be responsible for clinically significant drug interactions with compounds such as midazolam (excess sedation) and rifabutin (uveitis). They have recently been reported to cause peripheral lipodystrophy, which is characterised by fat redistribution, hypertension, hyperglycaemia, insulin resistance and possibly accelerated atherosclerosis. In light of this novel form of toxicity, their benefit–risk ratio needs to be re-evaluated.

1.17   B: Misoprostol

Warfarin, but not heparin, is associated with skeletal and central nervous system (CNS) defects if the fetus is exposed in the first trimester, while exposure during the third trimester increases the risk of intracranial haemorrhage during delivery. Misoprostol is associated with the Moebius syndrome. Diazepam, oral contraceptives and aspirin were initially thought to possess some terato-genic risk but formal cohort and case–control studies and meta-analyses have provided some evidence that these drugs are safe.

1.18   B: It is associated with a two-fold increased risk of breast cancer

Oestrogens should be combined with progestogens in patients with an intact uterus to reduce the risk of endometrial cancer, but can be used by themselves in patients who have had a hysterectomy. Hormone replacement therapy (HRT) has many benefits, including prevention of bone loss and possibly dementia, and the relief of menopausal symptoms. There are also many risks, including an increased risk of endometrial cancer (even in patients taking combined hormone therapy), breast cancer (approximately two-fold) and venous throm-boembolism. The beneficial effect of HRT on bone loss is more marked in patients who begin therapy within five years after the menopause. Raloxifene is a new non-steroidal selective oestrogen receptor modulator (SERM), which is just as effective as conventional forms of hormone replacement therapy. It has oestrogenic effects on bone and serum lipids, but does not stimulate endome-trial growth (ie it exerts an antioestrogenic effect). Preliminary findings suggest that it is also protective against breast cancer.

1.19   C: Activated charcoal reduces the enterohepatic circulation of drugs

Gastric lavage is best reserved for patients who present within 1 hour of an overdose, although with drugs which reduce gastric emptying, such as, anticholinergics, the time interval can be longer. Ipecacuanha syrup is associated with an increased risk of aspiration pneumonitis and oesophageal damage and should not be used. Haemodialysis is useful for drugs with a low volume of distribution (ie drugs such as aspirin which reside mostly within the plasma) and is not used for drugs with a high volume of distribution, such as tricyclic antidepressants. Forced alkaline diuresis should only be considered in very severe cases of aspirin poisoning.

1.20   B: Ciclosporin

Grapefruit juice contains compounds that are inhibitors of the cytochrome P450 isoform CYP3A4. The ability of grapefruit juice to inhibit drug metabolism was first shown with the calcium-channel blocker felodipine. Subsequent investigations have shown that grapefruit juice can interact with many CYP3A4 substrates, including terfenadine (leading to QT prolongation), cisapride (QT prolongation), ciclosporin (ciclosporin toxicity), and the protease inhibitors. The interaction with the protease inhibitors can in fact be used therapeutically to increase their bioavailability and so their effectiveness.

1.21   E: Genetically determined deficiencies of some of the drug metabolising enzymes have been described

Drug metabolism is conventionally divided into two phases – phase I and phase II. The main role of drug metabolism is to convert lipophilic compounds into hydrophilic metabolites, which can then be excreted from the body. Drug metabolism can also result in the formation of toxic metabolites that may be responsible for idiosyncratic toxicity. In addition, it can result in the formation of active metabolites, such as norfluoxetine in the case of fluoxetine. Phase I pathways are usually catalysed by cytochrome P450 enzymes, of which there are many different isoforms, while phase II pathways are catalysed by a number of enzymes, including glucuronyl transferase and *N*-acetyltransferase. Many of these enzymes can be either inhibited or induced and some also show genetically determined deficiencies. For example, fluoxetine is metabolised by the P450 isoform CYP2D6, which is deficient in 6–10% of the UK population. Metabolism occurs in all organs, apart from those of ectodermal origin. The liver is the main site; other sites include skin, gut wall, kidney, lungs and brain.

1.22   A: Less likely to cause parkinsonism

Typical neuroleptic drugs such as chlorpromazine have been used for many years in the treatment of schizophrenia. Their usefulness is limited by their propensity to cause extrapyramidal adverse effects. Atypical neuroleptics are less likely to cause extrapyramidal adverse effects. In addition, they affect not only the positive symptoms (like the typical neuroleptics), but also affect the negative symptoms, which are not improved by the typical neuroleptics. In comparison to the typical neuroleptics, the atypical neuroleptics are less likely to cause neuroleptic malignant syndrome and hyperprolactinaemia (except perhaps risperidone), but are more likely to induce weight gain. Atypical neuroleptics include clozapine, risperidone, olanzapine, sertindole and quetiapine.

1.23   E: Inhibition of GABA transaminase

Anticonvulsants often have more than one mode of action, although their efficacy can often be rationalised on the basis of one main mode of action. In general, the mode of action of anticonvulsants can be divided into one of three groups:

- Inhibition of sodium conductance: these include phenytoin, carbamazepine, sodium valproate and lamotrigine
- Enhancement of GABAergic action in the CNS: this may be secondary to binding to the GABA receptor (phenobarbital, benzodiazepines), inhibition of GABA transaminase (vigabatrin) or inhibition of GABA re-uptake (tiagabine)
- Miscellaneous: includes inhibition of calcium conductance (ethosuximide) and drugs such as gabapentin where the mode of action has not yet been determined.

1.24   C: It interacts with bendroflumethiazide (bendrofluazide)

Lithium is used for the treatment of bipolar depression and for the prophylaxis of unipolar depression. It does not affect mood in normal individuals. It is handled like sodium by the body and is excreted via the kidneys. Therefore, its use should be avoided in patients with moderate to severe renal impairment. It is also excreted in breast milk and its use should be avoided in breast-feeding mothers. It has a narrow therapeutic index, and its levels need to be monitored. Its renal excretion can be affected by non-steroidal anti-inflammatory drugs (NSAIDs) and diuretics, which can precipitate lithium toxicity. Adverse effects include goitre, hypothyroidism, tremor, convulsions and nephrogenic diabetes insipidus.

1.25   C: Atenolol

An acute attack of gout should be treated with high-dose NSAIDs or colchicine. Commencement of therapy for chronic gout with drugs such as allopurinol or uricosurics such as probenecid, if not covered by NSAIDs, can sometimes precipitate an acute attack. Aspirin and salicylates antagonise the uricosuric drugs and should therefore be avoided in patients with gout. Other drugs that can cause hyperuricaemia include diuretics, adenosine, ciclosporin, inosine pranobex, and alcohol.

1.26   E: Clarithromycin is active against atypical mycobacteria

Clindamycin penetrates bone well and is active against *Staphylococcus aureus*, which means it can be used in the treatment of osteomyelitis. It is particularly liable to cause pseudomembranous colitis. Methicillin-resistant *S. aureus* (MRSA or 'superbugs') have attracted media attention recently. In most cases, MRSA can be eliminated by topical therapy. Systemic therapy is only required when systemic infection is suspected: teicoplanin may be effective in such cases. Co-amoxiclav and flucloxacillin can cause cholestatic hepatitis, which can appear up to 6 weeks after stopping the drug. The liver toxicity is thought to be due to clavulanic acid rather than amoxicillin. Clarithromycin, a macrolide, is often used in HIV positive patients as prophylaxis against atypical mycobacteria.

1.27   D: It is treated with phenytoin

Digoxin is a drug with a narrow therapeutic index. Toxicity (even when levels are within the therapeutic range) can be precipitated by hypokalaemia, hypomagnesaemia and hypercalcaemia. Changes in the plasma sodium concentration have no effect on digoxin toxicity *per se*. Digoxin toxicity may manifest with symptoms such as nausea, vomiting, xanthopsia, or electrocardiogram (ECG) changes such as ST depression (reversed tick pattern) or cardiac arrhythmias. Phenytoin can be used to treat digoxin-induced cardiac arrhythmias.

1.28   B: It can only be used in amyotrophic lateral sclerosis

The cause of motor neurone disease (MND) is unknown. It has been postulated that excitotoxic neurotransmitters such as glutamate may be involved in the pathogenesis of MND. Riluzole antagonises the effects of glutamate on nerve cells by inhibiting its release and protecting cells from glutamate-mediated damage. It has been licensed 'to extend life or the time to mechanical ventilation for patients with amyotrophic lateral sclerosis'. It is not licensed for use in other forms of MND, such as progressive muscular atrophy and progressive bulbar palsy. Riluzole has a modest effect on mortality in patients with amyotrophic lateral sclerosis but there is no evidence that it improves either functional capacity or quality of life. Riluzole causes an elevation of liver enzymes in approximately 1% of patients.

1.29   E: Insulin receptors are linked to transmembrane protein tyrosine kinases

Drugs produce their actions by acting upon receptors, ion channels and enzymes. Most receptors are present on the plasma membrane, although oestrogen and steroid receptors are located within the cytosol and nucleus. Receptors interacting with G proteins can either modulate adenylate cyclase activity or activate phospholipase C. Insulin acts on cells by interacting with a receptor that has an extracellular hormone-binding domain and a cytoplasmic enzyme domain with protein tyrosine kinase activity. When tissues are continuously exposed to an agonist the numbers of receptors decrease or there is receptor desensitisation: this may cause tachyphylaxis (loss of efficacy with repeated doses).

1.30   C: Long-term therapy with omeprazole without antibiotics can alter the distribution of infection within the stomach

Patients with peptic ulcer who are infected with *Helicobacter pylori* have been shown to benefit from eradication therapy. However, there is little evidence that patients with non-specific dyspepsia will benefit from treatment with antibiotics. The use of antisecretory drugs in *H. pylori*-infected patients reverses the predominantly antral pattern of gastritis and increases the severity of corpus gastritis. The pattern of gastritis then resembles that more commonly associated with the development of mucosal atrophy. There is accumulating epidemiological evidence suggesting an association between *H. pylori* infection and cancer of the gastric corpus and antrum (but not of the duodenum). Eradication therapy, of which there are numerous regimens, generally has a success rate in excess of 90%.

1.31   C: It can lead to bone marrow suppression

Patients who are HCV-RNA positive with chronic hepatitis on biopsy should be considered for treatment with interferon-α. Normalisation of serum transaminases is seen in 50% of patients, but in half of these, transaminase levels rise again after stopping therapy. The sustained response rate is 15–25%; those individuals most likely to develop severe liver disease may be the least likely to respond to antiviral treatment. Treatment is contraindicated in patients with autoimmune disease, active psychiatric disorder, alcohol abuse, decompensated liver disease and pregnancy. Fever, headache and myalgia (which can be alleviated by pretreatment with paracetamol), anorexia and fatigue are common side-effects, while bone marrow suppression, alopecia, seizures, retinopathy and psychosis are more rare adverse effects.

1.32   A: Tinnitus

Tinnitus and deafness are seen in salicylate poisoning of any severity. Salicylates directly stimulate the respiratory centre to increase the depth and rate of respiration, causing a respiratory alkalosis. A variable degree of metabolic acidosis is also present because of the loss of bicarbonate. Increased tissue glycolysis and increased peripheral demand for glucose can cause hypoglycaemia. Salicylates have a warfarin-like action on the vitamin K1–epoxide cycle and can lead to hypoprothrombinaemia. Peptic ulceration is a feature of chronic salicylate therapy and not of acute poisoning.

1.33   E: It has an insidious onset

Neuroleptic malignant syndrome is an idiosyncratic reaction to therapeutic doses of phenothiazines, thioxanthines or butyrophenones. It develops insidiously over 1 to 3 days, and is characterised by hyperthermia, muscle rigidity, impaired consciousness and tachycardia and elevated creatine phosphokinase (CPK) levels. Dantrolene, but not calcium-channel blockers, may be of value. The mechanism responsible for the condition is unknown.

1.34   D: Propafenone has β-adrenoceptor-blocking activity

Adenosine is of little use in atrial fibrillation. Digoxin toxicity can lead to most types of arrhythmias, including atrial fibrillation. Digoxin is of use in chronic atrial fibrillation but not in paroxysmal atrial fibrillation. Sotalol has both class II and class III anti-arrhythmic properties, and can be used in both ventricular and supraventricular tachycardias. Propafenone is a class Ic drug with actions on sodium channels, calcium channels and β-blocking activity. QT-interval prolongation may lead to *torsades de pointes,* which is difficult to treat with other anti-arrhythmics, but may respond to magnesium. Magnesium has no effect on atrial fibrillation.

1.35   A: Rifabutin and clarithromycin

Zidovudine and aciclovir are often used together in patients with AIDS without causing any harmful effects. Aspirin and streptokinase were shown in the ISIS-2 study to have a beneficial effect in patients with acute myocardial infarction. Naproxen and penicillamine are often used together in patients with rheumatoid arthritis. Rifabutin metabolism can be inhibited by clarithromycin, which may result in anterior uveitis. Atenolol is commonly used together with isosorbide mononitrate in patients with angina.

1.36   B: All serious ADRs should be reported

The spontaneous adverse drug reaction (ADR) reporting scheme in the UK is called the yellow card scheme. Reporting is voluntary; it is recommended that all serious ADRs and all ADRs to new drugs (marked by ▼ in the *BNF*) should be reported. Doctors, dentists, coroners and, more recently, pharmacists are allowed to report on yellow cards. It has been estimated that only 10% of all serious ADRs and 3–4% of all ADRs are actually reported: such gross under-reporting means that the yellow card data cannot be used to estimate the frequency of a particular ADR. Yellow card reports provide a signal that a drug may have the propensity to cause a particular ADR: this can provide the impetus to initiate further epidemiological studies to allow a causal relationship to be established between an ADR and a drug.

1.37   E: Vd can be calculated from a knowledge of the dose and concentration in plasma if the drug demonstrates linear kinetics

Distribution volume is the volume of fluid in which the drug appears to distribute with a concentration equal to that in plasma. It can be calculated from knowledge of the dose and concentration as long as the drug demonstrates linear kinetics. For example, for a drug that remains within the circulation, the distribution volume will be similar to the blood volume, ie five litres. The distribution volume can be significantly higher than that of body water if the drugs are distributed mainly within peripheral tissues. For example, the volume of distribution of chloroquine is 13 000 litres. Drugs with a low Vd, such as aspirin, are mainly within the plasma and so can be removed by haemodialysis, particularly in overdose situations.

1.38   D: Iodide can cause goitre in euthyroid patients

The mainstay of treatment of thyrotoxicosis is the thioamides (carbimazole and propylthiouracil). Both inhibit the iodination of tyrosine and coupling of iodotyrosines. In addition, propylthiouracil, but not carbimazole, inhibits the peripheral conversion of T_4 to T_3. It usually takes 4 to 8 weeks for these drugs to have an effect. In that time, β-blockers are useful: they block the adrenergic effects of excess thyroid hormone, such as sweating and tremor, but have no effect on basal metabolic rate. In euthyroid subjects an excess of iodide from any source can cause goitre. Radioactive iodine emits mainly β radiation (90%), which penetrates only 0.5 mm of tissue. It does emit some of the more penetrating gamma rays, which can be detected with a Geiger counter.

1.39   E: Ethanol prevents methanol toxicity by inhibiting its oxidation within the liver

Methanol is eliminated in humans by oxidation to formaldehyde, formic acid and carbon dioxide. This is catalysed by the enzyme alcohol dehydrogenase. Blurred vision with a clear sensorium occurs 8–36 hours after poisoning, although optic atrophy is a late finding. Blood methanol levels should be determined as soon as possible. Methanol levels in excess of 50 mg/dl are thought to be an absolute indication for haemodialysis and ethanol treatment. The latter inhibits methanol oxidation by competing for alcohol dehydrogenase. Patients with methanol poisoning usually have a metabolic acidosis with an elevated anion gap.

1.40   D: Metronidazole

Drugs that inhibit the oxidation of acetaldehyde can cause a systemic reaction if taken with alcohol. This is the basis for the use of disulfiram as aversive treatment for alcoholism. Metronidazole can also inhibit acetaldehyde oxidation and tinidazole may have the same effect. Other drugs that can lead to flushing with alcohol include procarbazine, chlorpropamide, ketoconazole and cefamandole. Naltrexone is used in the treatment of alcoholics.

1.41   A: Weaker inhibitors of thrombin

Low-molecular-weight heparins (LMWHs) have mean molecular weights in the range of 4–6 kDa. Compared to unfractionated heparin (UFH), they are weaker inhibitors of thrombin (factor IIa), but inhibit the coagulation enzyme Xa to a similar extent. Elimination of LMWHs is mainly via the kidneys and is therefore likely to be reduced in patients with renal failure. Current evidence suggests that the risk of bleeding is similar with both sets of compounds. Immune-mediated thrombocytopenia occurs with both LMWH and UFH; the risk may be lower with LMWH although this needs to be confirmed in larger studies. The osteopenic effect of LMWH may be less than that of UFH.

1.42 B: Corticosteroid replacement is necessary in patients on aminoglutethimide

In postmenopausal women, peripheral tissues are the main site of oestrogen production, usually by conversion of androstenedione and testosterone by aromatase to oestrone and estradiol. These extraglandular sites of oestrogen production can be inhibited by aromatase inhibitors. Aminoglutethimide was the first of these inhibitors but was rather non-specific, causing inhibition of adrenal cortical enzymes as well. This necessitated the use of corticosteroid replacement. Anastrozole is a new-generation aromatase inhibitor that is more potent and highly selective. As a result it does not affect adrenal function.

1.43 B: Heart valve regurgitation has been shown to be associated with treatment with fenfluramine and phentermine

Various drugs have been used for the treatment of obesity with varying degrees of success. Appetite suppressants such as fenfluramine and phentermine have been associated with primary pulmonary hypertension and, more recently, with valvular heart disease. Although the prevalence of aortic and mitral regurgitation has varied in different studies, there is a consensus that these appetite suppressants lead to valvular heart disease (regurgitation rather than stenosis). The mechanism is unknown but may be related to increased production of serotonin (akin to the valve lesions seen in carcinoid syndrome). There is no evidence at the time of publication of this book that selective serotonin reuptake inhibitors (SSRIs) (which are used for treatment of obesity) also lead to valvular heart disease. Sibutramine is a relatively new antiobesity agent that increases blood pressure – frequent monitoring is required in patients; because of this it is also contraindicated in patients with hypertension.

1.44 A: Trazodone

Priapism is a prolonged and painful erection that cannot be relieved by sexual fulfilment. It has been reported in association with:

- phenothiazines, including chlorpromazine, promazine and fluphenazine
- the butyrophenone haloperidol
- trazodone but not conventional tricyclic antidepressants
- α-adrenoceptor antagonists, including prazosin, phenoxybenzamine and labetalol

- warfarin
- intracavernosal papaverine.

1.45   C: Desferrioxamine

The following antidotes can be used in patients with acute poisoning:

oral anticoagulants	vitamin K
benzodiazepines	flumazenil
β-blockers	atropine
	glucagon
carbon monoxide	oxygen
cyanide	oxygen
	dicobalt edetate
	hydroxocobalamin
	sodium thiosulphate
	sodium nitrite
digoxin	digoxin-specific antibody fragments
ethylene glycol	ethanol
	fomepizole
ferrous sulphate/	
fumarate and other salts	desferrioxamine
methanol	ethanol
opioids	naloxone
organophosphates	atropine
	pralidoxime
paracetamol	N-acetylcysteine

1.46   B: Decrease in gut motility

Stimulation of the α-adrenoceptor leads to vasoconstriction of most vessels in the body, in particular in the skin, mucosae, abdominal viscera and coronary circulation. Further actions include decrease in gut motility, contraction of the pregnant uterus, and decreased exocrine secretion by pancreatic acini and contraction of the radial muscle of the iris. Cholinergic activity and nitric oxide are largely responsible for penile erection.

1.47   C: Increased release of virus from cells

Zanamivir is a neuraminidase inhibitor, and is licensed for the treatment of influenza A or B within 48 hours of the onset of symptoms. Neuraminidase in the virus breaks down N-acetylneuraminic acid in respiratory secretions; this allows the virus to penetrate the surfaces of cells. Inhibition of the neuraminidase prevents infection and, in some cases, complications such as otitis media. Neuraminidase is also necessary for the optimal release of virus from infected cells, an action that increases the spread of virus and the intensity of the infection. Inhibition of neuraminidase decreases the likelihood of illness and reduces the severity of any illness that does develop. Zanamivir is inhaled through the mouth; the majority of the drug ends up in the oropharynx; overall, the drug is only 10–20% bioavailable. Zanamivir can decrease bronchial airflow, and should be used with caution in patients with chronic respiratory disease in whom it can induce clinically significant bronchospasm.

1.48   B: Can cause neutropenia and thrombocytopenia

Cephalosporins, like the penicillins, have a β-lactam ring. There is therefore a 20% risk of cross-sensitivity between the two groups: if a patient has had a severe reaction to penicillin such as anaphylaxis, then cephalosporins should either not be used at all or with extreme caution. Most cephalosporins have half-lives less than 3 hours. Cephalosporins are associated with a number of adverse effects, including skin rashes, anaphylaxis, neutropenia and thrombocytopenia, and are one of the most important causes of *Clostridium difficile* diarrhoea. Indeed, the current epidemic of *C. difficile* diarrhoea has been blamed on the British Thoracic Society guidelines that recommended the use of cephalosporins in the treatment of community-acquired pneumonia.

1.49   D: Sarcoidosis

The hypercalcaemia of sarcoidosis responds to steroids better than the other causes listed. Irrespective of the cause of hypercalcaemia, the first choice of treatment should always be rehydration with normal saline. Furosemide (frusemide) used concomitantly does not provide a better calcium-reducing effect. Only when patients have been rehydrated should bisphosphonates be used.

1.50   A: Approximately 8% of the population cannot convert codeine to morphine

Morphine is the drug of choice for controlling severe forms of pain. It is available in various formulations, including:

- Normal-release preparation: onset of action 20 minutes; peak drug levels 60 minutes
- Twice-daily controlled-release preparations: onset of action 1–2 hours; peak drug levels at 4 hours

- Once-daily controlled-release preparation: slower onset of action with peak drug levels at 8.5 hours.

Both diamorphine and codeine are pro-drugs, being converted to morphine in the body. Diamorphine is more soluble than morphine. Codeine is converted to morphine by the P450 enzyme CYP2D6, which is polymorphically expressed, being absent in 8–10% of the population. Many of the effects of morphine are subject to the phenomenon of tolerance, including the analgesic and euphoric effects. Importantly, miosis is not subject to tolerance and can be used as a sign to indicate opiate misuse.

1.51   C: Drugs with intrinsic sympathomimetic activity are less likely to cause bradycardia

Beta-blockers have many different properties, which can be used to differentiate their actions and side-effect profile. These include lipophilicity, cardioselectivity and intrinsic sympathomimetic activity (ISA). Beta-blockers with ISA are less likely to cause bradycardia. Beta-blockers such as atenolol are cardioselective but not cardiospecific: this means that they can still affect $\beta2$ receptors, especially when used in high dosage. Beta-blockers have class II anti-arrhythmic properties and, apart from sotalol (which also has class III properties), are unlikely to affect the QT interval. Celiprolol is a 'vasodilating' β-blocker and usually decreases total peripheral resistance. Esmolol is a short-acting β-blocker that is given intravenously to treat supraventricular arrhythmias.

1.52   A: Can cause selective IgA deficiency

Phenytoin is an anticonvulsant used for the treatment of generalised tonic–clonic convulsions and partial seizures. It can exacerbate myoclonic epilepsy, and can precipitate seizures when levels are high. It displays zero-order kinetics, ie due to saturation of metabolism; small changes in dose can lead to disproportionate increase in serum levels, with dose-dependent toxicity. It can cause a wide variety of adverse effects, including immune-mediated adverse reactions such as skin rashes, hepatitis and aplastic anaemia. It can also lead to other immunological abnormalities affecting both the cellular and humoral arms of the immune system. With respect to the latter, selective IgA deficiency is a well-recognised adverse reaction. Phenytoin is an enzyme inducer and can cause vitamin D deficiency, leading to osteomalacia. Phenytoin is also an anti-arrhythmic, used to treat digoxin-induced arrhythmias. It can, however, also lead to rhythm abnormalities such as bradycardia and ectopic beats in 2% of patients.

1.53   A: Cimetidine and dapsone

Rifampicin is an enzyme inducer, which can lower ciclosporin levels, leading to graft rejection. This is a serious interaction that can be overcome by monitoring ciclosporin levels and increasing the dose. Cimetidine is an enzyme inhibitor that can inhibit phenytoin metabolism, leading to phenytoin toxicity. Ritonavir is a potent enzyme inhibitor: it can inhibit the metabolism of fluoxetine, which can lead to a potentially fatal reaction called the serotonin syndrome. Erythromycin is an enzyme inhibitor that can affect the metabolism of cisapride: this can lead to prolongation of the QT interval and occasionally to *torsades de pointes* and sudden death. Cimetidine is an enzyme inhibitor that is known to inhibit dapsone metabolism. However, it results in reduced formation of a toxic metabolite of dapsone: this toxic metabolite is known to cause methaemoglobinaemia. This combination has therefore been used in patients with dermatitis herpetiformis to improve the tolerability of dapsone.

1.54   D: Rivastigmine binds to both the anionic and esteratic sites of the enzyme

Alzheimer's disease is characterised by decreased acetylcholine activity, and currently available drugs aim to increase cholinergic activity. Acetylcholine is broken down by acetylcholinesterase (AChE), and inhibition will increase acetylcholine activity. AChE has both anionic and esteratic sites; its activity can be inhibited by binding to either site. Donepezil and the recently withdrawn drug tacrine both act at the anionic site in a reversible fashion: they so have a relatively short duration of enzyme inhibition. However, donepezil has a long half-life (70 hours) and so only needs to be dosed once daily. Metrifonate, a pro-drug, which is converted to an active metabolite that binds irreversibly to the esteratic site of AChE, was recently withdrawn because of its potential to cause respiratory paralysis. Like acetylcholine, rivastigmine binds to both the anionic and esteratic sites; it needs to be administered twice daily.

1.55   E: Vigabatrin–anterior uveitis

Cerivastatin is an HMG-CoA reductase inhibitor that is highly potent, but causes rhabdomyolysis to a greater extent than the other HMG-CoA reductase inhibitors. For this reason, it was withdrawn from the market. Indinavir is a protease inhibitor that can crystallise out in urine, particularly when concentrations in plasma are high, and may in some cases lead to renal stones. Tolcapone is a catechol-*O*-methyltransferase (COMT) inhibitor used in Parkinson's disease; it was withdrawn because of its potential to cause hepatotoxicity and neuroleptic malignant syndrome but it is to be re-introduced soon for resistant patients who have not responded to entacapone. Vigabatrin causes peripheral visual field constriction in 30% of patients. This is thought to be irreversible, and although the mechanism of the adverse effect is not known, the retina is thought to be the site of toxicity. Pergolide is a dopamine agonist, and like all drugs of this class, it can cause fibrotic reactions, including pulmonary fibrosis, pleural fibrosis and retroperitoneal fibrosis.

1.56   E: It inhibits purine synthesis

Leflunomide is a disease-modifying antirheumatic drug, like gold, penicilla-mine, chloroquine, ciclosporin, sulfasalazine, methotrexate and azathioprine. Leflunomide inhibits pyrimidine synthesis through inhibition of dihydro-orotate dehydrogenase, and is rapidly converted to an active metabolite. Its efficacy is comparable to that of sulfasalazine and methotrexate.

1.57   B: Dose requirements are genetically determined

Warfarin is an oral anticoagulant, which acts as a vitamin K antagonist by inhibiting vitamin K epoxide reductase. Dose requirements vary widely: these are at least partly determined by genetic polymorphisms affecting the P450 enzymes (CYP2C9) responsible for the metabolism of warfarin. The dose can be adjusted by monitoring the international normalised ratio (INR). Overdosage predisposes to bleeding, which can be treated with fresh frozen plasma and vitamin K. Warfarin does not affect bone density; however, osteoporosis can be caused by heparin.

1.58   A: Accidental injection of lidocaine (lidocaine) into the systemic circulation may increase myocardial and neuronal excitability

Lidocaine, an amide local anaesthetic, is commonly used for minor surgery and in dental practice. Its duration of action can be prolonged by the addition of adrenaline (epinephrine), which causes vasoconstriction. Lidocaine is short-er acting than bupivacaine, and undergoes extensive metabolism. Intravenous injection can lead to cardiac arrhythmias and seizures.

1.59   D: The incidence of benign breast disease may be increased

Oral contraceptives contain progestogens, which inhibit luteinising hormone (LH) release, while the oestrogen component inhibits follicle stimulating hormone (FSH) release. Oestrogens, particularly at high dosage, promote blood clotting: this risk is increased in women over 35 years, who are obese and smokers. Third-generation oral contraceptives have a two-fold higher risk of venous thromboembolism than second-generation compounds. Thrombogenicity is also increased in patients who are carriers of the factor V Leiden mutation. There is also a small increase in the absolute risk of stroke with the oral contraceptive. The oral contraceptive pill also has many beneficial effects, including a reduced risk of benign breast disease and of ovarian cancer.

1.60 A: Does not have a beneficial effect if administered at the time of the first ever demyelinating event

Interferon-β has demonstrated benefits in the treatment of patients with established multiple sclerosis, including slowing the progression of physical disability, reducing the rate of clinical relapses, and reducing the development of brain lesions, as assessed by magnetic resonance imaging (MRI), and brain atrophy. A recent study has shown that initiating treatment at the time of the first demyelinating event is beneficial in patients with lesions on MRI that indicate a high risk of clinically definite multiple sclerosis.

ANSWERS

Endocrinology

ENDOCRINOLOGY: 'BEST OF FIVE'

2.1   C: Sick euthyroidism

These thyroid function tests are not typical of either prir
(TSH should be raised) or secondary hypothyroidism (TS┌ ┴┴┴,
but Free T_4 should be low). In the clinical context, 'sick euthyroidism' (sometimes referred to as changes of non-thyroidal illness) is the most likely explanation. In generally ill patients, T_3 levels fall first (within 24 hours) as T_4 to T_3
conversion is rapidly inhibited. Free T_4 levels may actually rise as a result. TSH
may then fall and occasionally becomes undetectable. A fall in free T_4 levels is
the last change to be seen. Drug interference would not typically cause a low
TSH and there is no need to invoke laboratory error in this case, as the changes
are typical of 'sick euthyroidism'. To avoid confusion and misdiagnosis, it is
generally advisable not to check thyroid function on in-patients unless there is
a very clear clinical indication.

2.2   D: To have a fine needle aspiration of the nodule for cytology

Around 90–95% of isolated thyroid nodules are benign adenomas or cysts.
However, the remainder may be malignant and can occur at any age. Papillary
thyroid cancer is the commonest thyroid tumour and has a very good prognosis
(up to 90% 10-year survival or more depending on the stage). Follicular thyroid
cancer has a less good prognosis and medullary thyroid cancer, which has a
much worse prognosis, may also present in this way. Anaplastic thyroid cancer
usually occurs in the elderly and progresses rapidly as a diffusely infiltrating
mass in the neck. Further investigation is necessary for euthyroid nodules. If the
patient is euthyroid, the nodule will usually be 'cold' in radionucleotide
scanning and this does not advance the diagnosis. Partly cystic nodules can be
malignant and ultrasound cannot rule out a malignancy. Malignancies can also
occur in multi-nodular glands. Thyroxine suppression results in inappropriate
delay and is not usually diagnostic. The patient should proceed to fine needle
aspiration (FNA) biopsy by an experienced operator and cytologist.

2.3   B: To encourage him to pursue a diet and exercise programme

This man has impaired fasting glucose (IFG – result between 6 and 7 mmol/l).
To diagnose impaired glucose tolerance (IGT) requires an oral glucose tolerance test to determine whether the 2-hour blood sugar after 75 g of glucose is
between 8 and 11 mmol/l. Most, but not all people with IFG also have IGT and
the conditions are very similar. Patients with IFG/IGT do not need screening for
microvascular complications (eyes, kidneys, feet) but are at the same high
cardiovascular risk as people who have diabetes (2-hour blood sugar > 11

mol/l). There is a risk of 30–50% over the next 5 years of progressing to true type 2 diabetes. Metformin reduces the risk of progression to IGT by 28% whereas diet and exercise resulted in a > 50% reduction in the number who progressed to diabetes in two recent studies.

2.4   C: To ask him to set his alarm clock for 0300 h to test his blood sugar on two occasions

Nocturnal fits in an insulin-treated patient are most likely to be hypoglycaemia unless proved otherwise. It is important to make the diagnosis before labelling the patient as epileptic and beginning anticonvulsant therapy that may be unnecessary, and 0300 h capillary blood sugar testing is a good way to do this. If the value is < 4.0 mmol/l then hypoglycaemia is a very possible cause of the fits. His morning low values are suggestive of night-time hypos, while the higher ones may be a recovery response to hypoglycaemia earlier in the night. If confirmed, the isophane insulin is most likely to blame and many diabetologists would change the long-acting insulin to a newer analogue such as insulin levemir or glargine, which have smoother profiles.

2.5   B: Patients with hepatocyte nuclear factor (HNF)-1 alpha mutations causing maturity-onset diabetes of the young (MODY-3) can be very successfully treated with sulphonylurea drugs

Up to 30% of patients with type 2 diabetes will currently fail oral medication and require insulin at some time due to progressive beta cell failure. Newer treatments with thiazolidinediones and glycolipoprotein (GLP)-1 agonists are hoped to reverse this trend and trials are in progress. Weight loss is beneficial at any stage and major weight loss (eg after gastric banding surgery) may in some cases result in reversal from diabetes to impaired glucose tolerance or even normoglycaemia. Raised liver enzymes (especially transaminases) are common due to hepatic fat deposits in the liver and toxicity (non-alcoholic steatohepatosis – NASH). The common lipid abnormality is low high density lipoprotein (HDL) and raised triglyceride levels rather than raised total cholesterol. Patients with diabetes due to HNF-1 alpha mutations (rare) are unusually sensitive to sulphonylureas.

2.6   A: Aortic root rupture is an important cause of death

Turner's syndrome is associated with the XO karyotype but partial deletions of the X chromosomes can also result in a similar though milder phenotype. Some girls are XO/XX mosaics and can develop spontaneous periods and even (very rarely) become pregnant. A related phenotype (web neck, short stature, wide-spaced nipples, cardiac defects) can be seen in Noonan's syndrome, which is an autosomal dominant condition and hence can affect boys. The X chromosome is normal. The phenotype in Turner's girls is often apparent at birth (web/ short neck, nail change, lymphoedema) and is an important diagnosis to make so that growth hormone therapy can be initiated early for maximal final height (growth hormone improves but does not normalise short stature at twice normal replacement doses) as well as screening for other major abnormalities including cardiac and renal abnormalities and deafness. Aortic root dilatation and rupture is increasingly recognised as an important cause of death and routine imaging is recommended in adulthood.

2.7 A: Blood glucose should be measured as a markedly raised level may account for the hyponatraemia

In the evaluation of hyponatraemia, a low serum osmolality is expected. A normal level should prompt a search for 'pseudohyponatraemia' in which dilution is caused by elements that are not measured in osmolality assessment – notably hypertriglyceridaemia and hyperproteinaemia. Hyperglycaemia is an important cause of dilutional hyponatraemia with low osmolality. The syndrome of inappropriate ADH secretion is common but can only be diagnosed with confidence in the presence of normal renal, adrenal and thyroid (exclude hypothyroidism) function, in the absence of diuretic therapy and in the presence of euvolaemia and sodium in the urine (suggesting that the patient is sodium replete). Low urine sodium (< 10 mmol/l) and hypovolaemia suggest body sodium loss, eg through vomiting, diarrhoea or fistula losses. Hypoadrenalism is an important life threatening cause of hyponatraemia with hypovolaemia in which sodium is present in the urine. Especially in pituitary disease (in which the renin–angiotensin–aldosterone system remains intact) it can occur in the absence of hyperkalaemia.

2.8 E: Occult use of purgatives is a possible cause if the urine potassium is low

The investigation of hypokalaemia is different in the normotensive to the hypertensive patient. Causes with a normal blood pressure include diuretic use or abuse, purgative abuse (K^+ lost in gastrointestinal (GI) tract and hence this is a cause with a low urinary potassium), thyrotoxicosis with periodic paralysis, Bartter syndrome or other tubular defects or Gittelman's syndrome. Gittelman's syndrome is the most common in the absence of any other features and a low magnesium level helps to confirm the diagnosis. Conn's syndrome, Liddle's syndrome, excess liquorice consumption or other causes of 'apparent mineralocorticoid excess' are possible causes if the patient is hypertensive.

2.9   C: Leptin is important in the timing of puberty

In recent years adipose tissue has been recognised to be an active endocrine organ secreting hormones that include leptin, adiponectin, resistin and visfatin. Leptin physiology is the best characterised. Leptin levels increase with increases in body weight and leptin acts on the hypothalamus to reduce appetite, but is probably most important as a signal to indicate adequate fat stores to allow the onset of puberty in girls. Adiponectin reduces insulin resistance.

2.10   B: The heights of both parents should be measured

Short stature in boys is commonly associated with delayed puberty (no onset of puberty by 14 years of age) even at this age. Mid-parental height should be calculated, as the boy may not be particularly short for his family. Systemic illness causing delayed puberty and short stature is not always apparent and important occult causes include hypothyroidism, Crohn's/coeliac disease and renal disease. Chromosomal analysis for short stature is mandatory in girls (to exclude Turner's syndrome) but unlikely to be informative in boys. A pineal hamartoma is a classical cause of precocious puberty.

2.11   D: The insulin receptor complex can acquire enzymatic function

The insulin receptor is part of the class of receptor tyrosine kinases in which once the ligand is bound, the receptor acts by enzymatically phosphorylating other proteins, triggering a cascade of proteins phosphorylating other proteins ('kinase cascade'). The molecular cause of insulin resistance in type 2 diabetes is unknown except in the less than 1% of cases with monogenic diabetes (maturity onset diabetes of the young). Insulin does not act via cyclic AMP. The insulin receptor is plasma membrane bound and does not migrate into the nucleus.

2.12   C: Sampling of ACTH from the draining venous plexus of the pituitary may be required

Once Cushing's syndrome is established (by overnight dexamethasone or urinary free cortisol testing), additional tests are required to distinguish the three main causes: a pituitary tumour (Cushing's disease); an adrenal adenoma/carcinoma; or ectopic ACTH, often from a bronchial adenoma, which may be too small to see even on high resolution computed tomography (CT) of the chest. Suppression in the high dose dexamethasone test suggests a pituitary adenoma and in this situation the ACTH is often in the 'normal' range, though of course this is not the 'normal' level you would expect to see in the presence of large amounts of circulating cortisol. Distinguishing a bronchial adenoma (ectopic ACTH) from pituitary disease especially when both are too small to see on scanning can be difficult. In this situation, CRH (corticotrophin releasing hormone) stimulation can be valuable as pituitary dependent disease tends to show a rise in ACTH and petrosal sinus sampling can show that the ACTH level draining the gland is very much higher than in the periphery, confirming the pituitary as the site of disease.

2.13   B: She must convert onto insulin therapy

As the population becomes more overweight, the number of individuals with type 2 diabetes becoming pregnant is increasing markedly – currently around 25% of all diabetic pregnancies. Unfortunately, almost all the tablet therapies for glucose lowering, blood pressure and cholesterol lowering are contra-indicated in pregnancy and have to be stopped. Mothers must convert to insulin therapy if they cannot be controlled on diet alone. Outcomes of pregnancy are as bad or possibly worse than in type 1 diabetes. Microalbuminuria frequently progresses to proteinuria during pregnancy and involvement of a renal physician may be required.

2.14   B: A pituitary tumour can usually be seen on magnetic resonance imaging (MRI) scanning

In the vast majority of cases, acromegaly is caused by a pituitary tumour and this is easily visible on MRI scanning (in contrast to tumours causing Cushing's syndrome for example). Prolactin is often co-secreted and moderately raised levels may be present. Diagnosis is made by failure to suppress growth hormone levels during a glucose tolerance test and a raised IGF-1 level is usually present. Treatment reduces sweating and some soft tissue swelling, but the majority of the acromegalic features do not resolve. An increase in both colonic polyps (adenomatous, premalignant) and colon cancer is reported and routine colonoscopy of patients with active disease is often recommended.

2.15   D: It is synthesised in the hypothalamus

Antidiuretic hormone (ADH) (vasopressin) is synthesised in the hypothalamus and transported via axons to the posterior pituitary. It is a cyclic nonapeptide that, although it is stored bound to neurophysin, circulates in the blood mostly in the unbound form. Its release is promoted by carbamazepine (resulting in 'inappropriate ADH syndrome') and is suppressed by alcohol.

2.16   D: Lithium therapy

Failure of secretion of antidiuretic hormone (ADH) results in cranial diabetes insipidus (DI), whereas tubular resistance to ADH action underlies the nephrogenic form. Untreated, dehydration results in a raised serum sodium, but the condition is not fatal in conscious individuals with access to water, as the thirst mechanism drives the individual to drink as required. Lithium, hypercalcaemia, hypokalaemia and drugs (including demeclocycline) inhibit the action of ADH and result in nephrogenic DI. Nephrogenic DI can be inherited in a sex-linked form and is paradoxically ameliorated to some degree by thiazide diuretics.

2.17   C: Exclusion of treatment with antiemetic drugs

Galactorrhoea is invariably the result of excess prolactin or increased sensitivity to it. It should not be confused with gynaecomastia in men, which is associated with increased oestrogen action. Gynaecomastia should prompt a search for chronic liver disease, hypogonadism or an oestrogen/human chorionic gonadotrophin (HCG)-producing occult malignancy of the lung or testis. Raised prolactin levels and galactorrhoea are frequently associated with dopamine-blocking drugs, especially major tranquillisers and antiemetics, but are rarely associated with antidepressants. If drug side-effects have been excluded, investigation involves thyroid function testing (rarely hypothyroidism induces hyperprolactinaemia via thyrotropin-releasing hormone (TRH)), a prolactin level and imaging of the pituitary. The latter is done because small or moderate elevations of prolactin can be caused by non-functioning and potentially sight-threatening tumours of the pituitary pressing on the pituitary stalk ('disconnection hyperprolactinaemia'). However, the commonest cause in premenopausal women is a prolactin microadenoma.

2.18   A: Elevated luteinising hormone (LH) levels

Anorexia is a 'stressed starvation' state with raised cortisol and growth hormone levels but low IGF-1 and a hypothalamic pattern of hypogonadism (low LH, follicle stimulating hormone (FSH) and oestrogen). Secondary amenorrhoea with axillary (but rarely pubic) hair loss is common but presentation earlier in childhood with primary amenorrhoea can occur.

2.19   A: Anosmia

Hypogonadism in a phenotypic man may be due to primary gonadal failure (typically Klinefelter's syndrome, karyotype XXY) with raised gonadotrophins (luteinising hormone (LH), follicle stimulating hormone (FSH)) or secondary gonadal failure with low LH and FSH. Causes of the latter include delayed puberty, pituitary damage or Kallman's syndrome (isolated LH/FSH failure, often with anosmia). Sex hormone binding levels are raised by oestrogen but reduced by androgen and hence tend to be relatively high in male hypogonadism. Exposure to androgens in utero can cause masculinisation of a female fetus but the result is usually intersex rather than a true phenotypic man.

2.20   D: Radioiodine may not be the ideal first-line treatment

The combination of hyperthyroidism and specific eye signs (other than simply lid retraction and lid lag) strongly suggests a diagnosis of primary hyperthyroidism due to Graves' disease. In this condition the thyroid is stimulated by antithyroid stimulating hormone (TSH) receptor agonist antibodies and TSH levels themselves are undetectably low. Antithyroid peroxidase antibodies are detectable in up to 90% of cases but these are not believed to be pathogenic. If the woman becomes pregnant, transplacental passage of agonist antibodies (not thyroxine itself, which has a shorter half-life and will be at normal levels after antithyroid drug treatment) can potentially result in neonatal thyrotoxicosis for several weeks although this is rare (around 4% of pregnancies with Graves' disease). In treatment, significant evidence suggests that radioiodine has a greater chance than other treatments of exacerbating the eye disease and should be deferred or given with steroid cover. Restoring euthyroidism rarely improves the eye manifestations and over-treatment (resulting in hypothyroidism) may actually make these worse.

2.21   C: Cardiomyopathy

Profound hypothyroidism is associated with a variety of neurological disturbances, including ataxia, deafness, paranoia, delusions and confusion ('myxoedema madness'). Autoimmune hypothyroidism is associated with an increased incidence of other autoimmune diseases, especially Addison's disease (Schmidt's syndrome) and vitiligo. Multiple serous effusions can occur and cardiac tamponade has been described as well as accelerated coronary artery disease, but cardiomyopathy is not a recognised feature.

2.22   E: Tenderness over the thyroid gland

Thyrotoxicosis due to Graves' disease, toxic multi-nodular goitre or toxic nodule rarely spontaneously remits. However, destructive thyroiditis due to subacute thyroiditis (also known as postviral, de Quervain's or granulomatous thyroiditis) spontaneously remits. This is associated with a short history, tenderness over the thyroid gland and a raised erythrocyte sedimentation rate (ESR) (sometimes confused with a viral sore throat), as well as absent uptake of radioiodine. This is usually followed by a period of transient hypothyroidism. Transient thyroiditis also occurs in the post-partum period and in patients with autoimmune thyroiditis (silent thyroiditis).

2.23   A: Amiodarone therapy

This pattern of thyroid function tests suggests thyrotoxicosis. It is also consistent with over-treatment or factitious ingestion of T_4, but not T_3 (as the latter would result in a low T_4 level). Hyperemesis gravidarum with very high human chorionic gonadotrophin (HCG) levels and the first trimester of pregnancy can result in mild thyrotoxicosis by crossreactivity between HCG and thyroid stimulating hormone (TSH) at the TSH receptor but HCG levels fall later in pregnancy. Systemic illness results initially in a low T_3 followed by a low TSH and in prolonged illness a low T_4; a raised free T_4 can occur but is unusual. Oestrogen and the oral contraceptive raise thyroxine binding globulin and total T_4 but not free T_4. Amiodarone therapy, however, can produce thyrotoxicosis or hypothyroidism, the former as a result of either iodine overload or a destructive thyroiditis, and can be difficult to treat. Hypothyroidism typically occurs in the first year of beginning amiodarone, but thyrotoxicosis can occur at any time.

2.24   C: Persistent generation of cyclic adenosine monophosphate (AMP)

G proteins are multi-molecular complexes that are characterised by their ability to hydrolyse guanosine triphosphate (GTP) to guanosine diphosphate (GDP) and are involved in many intracellular processes. In endocrinology they are activated by many membrane receptors (eg the receptors of adrenaline (β), thyroid stimulating hormone (TSH), luteinising hormone (LH), follicle stimulating hormone (FSH) and GHRH). G proteins themselves activate adenylate cyclase to generate cyclic AMP. In the process of activation, the α-subunit separates from the β- and γ-subunits but it then spontaneously hydrolyses GTP and reforms the α-β-γ trimer. Mutations in the G proteins have been described which prevent this spontaneous inactivation, causing persistent cyclic AMP generation and resulting in tumour formation (eg growth hormone (GH)-secreting tumours in acromegaly, but not non-functioning pituitary tumours) or gland overactivity (toxic thyroid nodule, McCune–Albright syndrome). Multiple endocrine neoplasia type II does not involve G proteins. G-protein abnormalities are associated with pseudohypoparathyroidism but not hypercalcaemia.

2.25   B: An adrenal carcinoma

This lady has Cushing's syndrome, confirmed by the raised 24-hour free cortisols. The short history is suggestive of an aggressive neoplastic process and the strong element of virilisation is suggestive of an adrenal carcinoma. This is further supported by the undetectable adrenocorticotrophic hormone (ACTH) levels as the cortisol from the neoplastic adrenal suppresses the pituitary. The prognosis is very poor in such cases. Cushing's syndrome is most commonly caused by an ACTH-secreting pituitary tumour but in this case, and in the case of ACTH production from a bronchial carcinoid, circulating ACTH levels would be detectable. Squamous cell carcinoma of the bronchus is rarely associated with Cushing's syndrome – the association is with small-cell lung cancer secreting ACTH. In the latter condition, the history is short but the biochemical features predominate (hypokalaemic alkalosis), ACTH levels are high, cushingoid features are typically absent, and extensive lung cancer is readily apparent on chest X-ray.

2.26   C: It causes vasodilatation

Atrial natriuretic peptide, as its name suggests, is a peptide hormone secreted from the myocardium that causes natriuresis (excretion of sodium). It is released under conditions of hypervolaemia (myocardial stretch) and its actions are all consistent with mechanisms to correct the hypervolaemic state: reduced thirst, vasodilatation and excretion of sodium. In the last mechanism it acts directly on the kidney rather than via suppression of aldosterone.

2.27   A: Fatigue

Glucocorticoid deficiency results in rather non-specific fatigue and weakness that responds within hours to glucocorticoid. Postural hypotension may also be a useful indicator but reflects more severe failure, as does hypoglycaemia. Salt craving and hyperkalaemia are manifestations of mineralocorticoid deficiency, which may co-exist.

2.28   A: A female infant will present with intersex

21-Hydroxylase deficiency accounts for around 95% of all congenital adrenal hyperplasia. Homozygous individuals may present with an addisonian crisis (salt losing in two-thirds of cases) in infancy (with hypotension) and in females may present as intersex due to the masculinising effect of excess androgen production from the affected adrenals. Intersex is not likely in boys, but premature puberty may occur. 17-OH progesterone is characteristically very high in this condition as it precedes the enzyme failure in the steroidogenic pathway.

2.29   A: A good response in terms of calcium levels to treatment with calcium and vitamin D

Idiopathic hypoparathyroidism is typically autoimmune in origin. It should be distinguished from pseudohypoparathyroidism, which is sometimes associated with short fourth and fifth metacarpals and in which resistance to parathyroid hormone (PTH) occurs, resulting in hypocalcaemia despite raised levels of PTH. Idiopathic hypoparathyroidism is associated with other autoimmune conditions (especially in autoimmune polyglandular failure type 1 where it is associated with mucocutaneous candidiasis, coeliac disease, and adrenal failure), but rarely with hyperthyroidism. It does respond well in terms of raising calcium levels to treatment with vitamin D and calcium. However, calcium levels should be maintained in the low–normal range to avoid hypercalciuria and renal stones. Tympanic membrane calcification is a manifestation of hypercalcaemia not hypocalcaemia.

2.30   C: Serum alkaline phosphatase reflects disease activity

Paget's disease is predominantly a condition of disordered bone turnover. Serum alkaline phosphatase is raised in more extensive cases and is a useful indicator of active disease and response to treatment. Standard treatment is with bisphosphonates–there is no place for treatment with vitamin D analogues. The disease is often asymptomatic and non-progressive. Indications for treatment include pain, impingement on joints, very high alkaline phosphatase (extensive disease), pressure effects (eg deafness) and high-output cardiac failure.

2.31   B: Hyperparathyroidism

MEN type 1 (MEN1) is associated with mutations in the gene *menin* and results in familial hyperparathyroidism, pituitary tumours and gastrointestinal (GI) neuroendocrine tumours (especially gastrinoma and insulinoma). The major morbidity comes from the GI tumours. There is also an increased incidence of carcinoid. MEN2 is associated with mutations in the *RET* proto-oncogene and results in hyperparathyroidism in association with medullary thyroid cancer and phaeochromocytoma. Both of the latter are potentially lethal.

2.32   A: A sulphonylurea screen

Spontaneous hypoglycaemia (not due to over-treatment of diabetes) should always be investigated. Serum insulin levels at the time of hypoglycaemia provide the most important information but C-peptide levels and a sulphonylurea screen on the same blood sample are also helpful. C-peptide and insulin levels are inappropriately high in insulinoma but these results are indistinguishable from occult sulphonylurea abuse. Factitious hypoglycaemia due to occult insulin administration would result in high insulin but not raised C-peptide levels. A glucose tolerance test is of no value in the investigation of fasting hypoglycaemia. Thyrotoxicosis is rarely associated with hypoglycaemia. Hypoadrenalism is, but 24-hour urinary free cortisol is a measure of glucocorticoid excess, not deficiency.

2.33   E: Yearly screening with urinary catecholamines in familial disease

Ten per cent of spontaneous phaeochromocytomas are malignant (less in familial disease), but this can only reliably be determined by the presence of local invasion or metastases. Tumour histology is often very dysplastic, even in lesions that subsequently follow a benign course, a feature common to many endocrine tumours. Malignant disease, when it occurs, is difficult to treat and is not radiosensitive. Benign tumours can also be fatal from hypertensive crises and cardiomyopathy, making it important to screen annually for new tumours in patients with familial disease (including MEN2). Initial treatment is with α-blockade before surgery (unopposed β-blockade can result in a hypertensive crisis). There is no association with islet cell tumours.

2.34   C: High gastrin levels area associated with pernicious anaemia

Although vasopressin has vasoconstrictive effects, the analogue DDAVP does not. Vasopressin secretion is increased by carbamazepine and other drugs that result in inappropriate ADH syndrome. Although administration of calcitonin lowers calcium levels, removal of the C-cells that make this hormone – as occurs with total thyroidectomy – does not appear to affect calcium homeostasis. The failure of acid secretion as seen in pernicious anaemia and with H_2^- or proton pump blockade does result in hypergastrinaemia. Glucagon levels are raised in diabetic ketoacidosis, but in long-standing disease the glucagon response to hypoglycaemia fails.

2.35   D: Withhold any antithyroid treatment and repeat thyroid function testing in 3 weeks

Thyrotoxicosis presenting in pregnancy is due either to Graves' disease or crossreactive activation of the thyroid stimulating hormone (TSH) receptor by the very high human chorionic gonadotrophin (HCG) levels in the first trimester of pregnancy (the two hormones have a common α-subunit). Characteristics of the latter condition are that it is commonly associated with hyperemesis gravidarum, occurs in the first trimester and subsides spontaneously in the subsequent weeks (as the HCG level falls), is biochemically mild, and is more frequently seen with twin or molar pregnancies. A confident diagnosis cannot be made in the absence of Graves' eye disease and a wait-and-see policy is appropriate if the degree of thyrotoxicosis is mild and the patient clinically well. Propylthiouracil may be used and is safe but is often unnecessary. Radionucleotide scans are contraindicated in pregnancy and subtotal thyroidectomy is only indicated in Graves' disease with ongoing thyrotoxicosis in patients intolerant of medication. There are no grounds for advising termination except in a molar pregnancy.

2.36   E: Short Synacthen testing followed by immediate treatment with hydrocortisone

External beam radiotherapy continues to cause pituitary damage for 20 years or more after treatment. It is most likely that this man has now developed panhypopituitarism with secondary gonadal failure, but also adrenal failure (low sodium and tiredness but the potassium is not raised as mineralocorticoid function is preserved in secondary adrenal failure) and possibly also secondary hypothyroidism (the thyroid stimulating hormone (TSH) is often misleadingly normal but T_4 testing shows a very low value). The most dangerous element here is adrenal failure. Insulin stress testing or treatment with thyroxine (which accelerates metabolism of adrenal steroids) may precipitate a fatal hypotensive crisis. Adrenal failure should be assumed. Short Synacthen testing (with synthetic adrenocorticotrophic hormone (ACTH) and cortisol sampling at 0, 30 and 60 minutes) is safe and if immediately available involves minimal delay. Alternatively, a sample for random cortisol could be saved before urgent treatment with parenteral hydrocortisone. Thyroxine and testosterone replacement can be commenced later.

2.37   D: Corticosteroids act more slowly because they act by modulating gene transcription

β-agonists like adrenaline act via cell surface 7-transmembrane receptors and once bound to their ligand activate G proteins that in turn activate the enzyme adenylcyclase. The result is rapid (seconds) generation of cyclic AMP, which acts as an intracellular second messenger to mediate the actions of the drug/hormone. Corticosteroids are lipid soluble but their effects are generated slowly because they act by modulating gene transcription and new proteins must either first be synthesised or existing ones be degraded. However, once generated, these changes in intracellular protein result in prolonged action beyond the serum half-life of the hormone.

2.38   B: A high renin and a high aldosterone level

Renal artery stenosis results in high renin and high aldosterone levels in contrast to Conn's syndrome in which the aldosterone is high but the renin is characteristically suppressed. While the aldosterone level is high in both cases, it will not discriminate between the two conditions.

2.39   E: 24-hour urinary free cortisol

To distinguish Cushing's syndrome from simple obesity, a 24-hour urinary free cortisol or an overnight low-dose (1 mg) dexamethasone suppression test is typically used. There is loss of diurnal variation in cortisol in Cushing's syndrome. This means that the morning cortisol remains high, but a high evening (midnight) value is strongly suggestive of organic disease. Salivary cortisol measurements can be used to assess this but the assay is not routinely available. Serum potassium is low and bicarbonate high in Cushing's syndrome but these features would also be seen in hypertension treated with a diuretic and are not very specific for Cushing's syndrome. Adrenocorticotrophic hormone (ACTH) levels may be inappropriately 'normal' in pituitary-dependent Cushing's syndrome. Adrenal or pituitary scanning may show abnormalities in Cushing's syndrome but in the absence of a biochemical diagnosis, radiological abnormalities could be due to non-functioning 'incidentalomas', which are relatively common at both sites.

2.40   B: Basal bolus insulin

The DIGAMI study shows that diabetics treated with intravenous insulin for at least the first 24 hours, followed by subcutaneous insulin for at least 3 months, have significantly lower mortality rates up to 3.4 years later. This is regardless of the form of treatment they were taking before the myocardial infarction (MI).

The mechanism of this is unclear but may be related to the reduction in free fatty acids released as part of the stress reaction. He has a degree of heart failure and renal impairment, meaning that metformin is contraindicated because of the risk of lactic acidosis and rosiglitazone because of heart failure. Acarbose at therapeutic doses is unlikely to achieve the benefits of insulin post-MI.

2.41   D: To reduce his insulin to maintain relatively high blood sugars (8–15 mmol/l) for at least 3 months

This individual has hypoglycaemia unawareness. This is relatively common in long-standing diabetics, particularly in individuals who have very tight blood sugar control and have frequent hypoglycaemic episodes. It appears that the recurrent hypos result in a blunting of the adrenaline (and glucagon) response to hypoglycaemia, making it harder for the individual to detect, take evasive action (eating) and avoid further hypos – hence the phrase 'hypos beget hypos'. A relaxation in diabetic control with reduced insulin doses for three months such that all hypoglycaemic episodes are avoided results in a restoration of hypoglycaemia awareness and is the most appropriate advice. While regular blood sugar testing may help, it is not sustainable in the long-term and will not in itself restore hypoglycaemia awareness. Eating every 2 hours may reduce hypoglycaemic episodes but would result in weight gain and would not be the ideal way to manage this problem.

2.42   B: Aggressive management of hypertension

At the stage of microalbuminuria in diabetic nephropathy, glomerular filtration rates are relatively well preserved and serum creatinine is normal. Aggressive hypertension management down to levels as low as 130/80 mmHg has proved to be the best method of delaying decline in renal function and progression to macroalbuminuria. Good glycaemic control is key to preventing the development of nephropathy in the first place but plays a rather minor role in preventing progression from micro- to macroalbuminuria. Likewise, a low protein diet and aggressive lipid lowering can contribute to maintaining renal function but their role is limited. Diuretics are not contraindicated in diabetic nephropathy and can be used to treat hypertension.

2.43 D: Trans-sphenoidal surgery

The best chance of cure of small- to moderate-sized growth-hormone-secreting pituitary tumours causing acromegaly is trans-sphenoidal surgery, with cure rates approaching 70% in experienced centres. With larger tumours, complete cure is unlikely, but it is still appropriate to debulk the tumour and follow with radiotherapy. Octreotide therapy is very effective at lowering growth hormone levels by inhibiting growth hormone synthesis and release. However, it is very expensive, has to be given parenterally at least monthly, does not effect a cure or cause much tumour shrinkage and its exact role in therapy remains to be defined. Only 20% of growth hormone (GH)-secreting tumours respond to bromocriptine, and yttrium implantation has now given way to the safer procedure of external beam radiotherapy via three overlapping fields.

2.44 C: Hydrocortisone 10 mg mane and 5 mg pm, and fludrocortisone 100 μg mane

In primary adrenocortical failure (Addison's disease) both gluco- and miner-alocorticoid (eg fludrocortisone) replacement therapy is essential. The gluco-corticoid treatment should be given at the lowest possible doses to avoid long-term hypercortisolaemia. Possible dosing for glucocorticoid replacement alone includes hydrocortisone 10 mg mane/5 mg pm, or 10 mg bd, predniso-lone 5 mg or dexamethasone 0.5 mg. Higher doses of any of these drugs, except in an emergency, are detrimental in the long-term, with cushingoid side-effects. Dexamethasone has no mineralocorticoid effect.

2.45 C: Prophylactic thyroidectomy and regular screening for phaeochromocytoma

Multiple endocrine neoplasia (MEN) type 2 comprises hypercalcaemia (hyper-parathyroidism) and two potentially fatal conditions: medullary thyroid cancer (MTC) and phaeochromocytoma. By the time MTC is detectable on thyroid imaging it is unlikely to be curable and patients positive on genetic testing are now being advised to have a prophylactic thyroidectomy, typically before the age of 10 years. Bilateral adrenalectomy is a more dangerous procedure and may miss extra-adrenal phaeochromocytomas. Hence routine adrenalectomy is not advised but urinary catecholamine secretion should be measured regularly (eg yearly) followed by imaging if the screen proves positive. Pituitary tumours are a feature of MEN1, not of MEN2.

2.46   A: A benign course is very likely in such cases

Scattered dark (terminal or non-vellus) facial hairs and an escutcheon (hair between the umbilicus and pubic area) are common in women, as is hair on the lower arms and legs. When associated with menstrual irregularity dating from soon after the menarche or early 20s, by far the most common diagnosis is polycystic ovarian syndrome. Normal or slightly raised levels of testosterone are typically present and a benign course with a 'plateau' in hair growth in the mid-20s is to be expected. Hair on the upper back is unusual. Signs of virilisation comprise clitoromegaly, voice deepening, breast atrophy, and male pattern baldness and indicate very marked increases in androgen levels. In such situations and whenever the testosterone level is markedly raised (eg > 5 nmol/l), screening for adrenal and ovarian tumours is mandatory. Congenital adrenal hyperplasia is also a cause but is usually diagnosed in childhood.

2.47   A: He should be started on a sulphonylurea, taught to test his own capillary glucose levels and be reassessed in 1 month

This gentleman is relatively thin and young and is likely to have type 1 diabetes. He will have some residual β cell function (insulin production) and in older individuals this may persist for several months or years. Weight loss at presentation is strongly suggestive of type 1 diabetes but does not always occur in this older age group. Urgent hospital admission is not necessary, as he is not ketotic or obviously unwell. However, he should be observed closely as his β cell function may decline rapidly. Metformin is not appropriate. Treatment with a sulphonylurea to augment insulin production seems reasonable in this case but the patient should be reviewed as soon as possible (eg in 1 month) in case it is proving ineffective or hypoglycaemia has been precipitated.

2.48   A: Amino acids are an increasingly important source of substrates for glucose synthesis

Liver glycogen supplies glucose in the first 12 hours of fasting but is rapidly used up. After this, amino acids are increasingly the source of glucose synthesis, as fatty acids cannot be converted to glucose. Significant protein breakdown and nitrogen losses result. Glucagon levels rise within the first 12 hours of starvation and remain high. Mild ketonuria is often detectable in the first 24 hours of starvation as the low insulin levels result in fatty acid mobilisation. At later stages of starvation, ketone bodies replace up to 50% of the brain's need for glucose, reducing the degree of protein breakdown required to fuel gluconeogenesis.

2.49   D: Treatment should commence with a statin

Such a high level of cholesterol in a young person without elevated triglyceride levels strongly suggests heterozygous familial hypercholesterolaemia (low-density lipoprotein (LDL) receptor defect). This is autosomal dominantly inherited and heterozygotes typically suffer myocardial infarction around the age of 40, consistent with this man's family history. Current treatment is with high doses of HMG-CoA reductase inhibitors. The addition of a fibrate or plasmapheresis is sometimes required and ezetimibe may be of value. Excess alcohol and uncontrolled diabetes are typically associated with a mixed (raised cholesterol and triglyceride) hyperlipidaemia.

2.50   C: Hyperparathyroidism and malignancy account for 90% of cases

Asymptomatic hypercalcaemia in women in this age group is typically due to hyperparathyroidism. Further investigation, particularly parathyroid hormone estimation, is required to rule out the possibility of malignancy (with bony metastases or parathyroid hormone-related protein production). Malignancy and hyperparathyroidism account for 90% of cases of chronic hypercalcaemia. Alkaline phosphatase levels may be raised in both conditions. 'Normal' or raised parathyroid hormone levels in the presence of hypercalcaemia confirm the diagnosis of hyperparathyroidism. In asymptomatic patients with hyperparathyroidism, the indications for parathyroidectomy are controversial but include calcium levels above 3.0 mmol/l, hypercalcaemic crisis and renal stones. Calcium levels are usually stable over many years and parathyroidectomy is frequently not required.

ANSWERS

Gastroenterology

GASTROENTEROLOGY: 'BEST OF FIVE' ANSWERS

3.1   E: The child should be offered vaccination against hepatitis B as soon as possible after birth

Hepatitis B is a hepatatrophic DNA virus that can cause both acute and chronic infection. Transmission can occur through blood-to-blood contact, unsafe sexual intercourse and by vertical transmission from mother to child. Infants have up to a 90% chance of becoming chronic hepatitis carriers if infected at birth and appropriate immunisation can prevent carrier status in up to 95% of cases. For this reason the Department of Health (DoH) recommends hepatitis screening for all pregnant women in the UK and that all children born to infected mothers be offered immunisation. In this case the mother is surface antigen positive confirming hepatitis B infection but e antigen negative with a low viral load indicative of chronic carrier status. In a woman from an area where hepatitis B is endemic, infection is likely to have occurred at birth. DoH guidelines suggest that infants born to mothers with high risks of transmission (acute infection during pregnancy, e antigen positive or high viral load) are given hepatitis B-specific immunoglobulin (HBIG) at birth. Infants born to women with low risks of transmission (e antigen negative, low viral load) should be offered vaccination against hepatitis B within 24 hours of birth with further doses at 1, 2 and 12 months. Immunity against hepatitis B should be confirmed at this time. Breast-feeding carries no risk of viral transmission to appropriately treated infants and should be actively encouraged.

3.2   E: Ursodeoxycholic acid will help her symptoms and may delay disease progression

Primary biliary cirrhosis has a peak incidence in the 5th decade and is characterised by portal inflammation and immune mediated destruction of the intra-hepatic bile ducts. Antimitochondrial antibodies are present in 90–95% of cases often before symptoms occur. Antibody titre does not correlate with disease activity however and is therefore not useful in determining prognosis or response to treatment. The commonest symptoms are of fatigue and pruritus (the cause of which is unclear and often unresponsive to treatment). Osteo-porosis and hyperlipidaemia are often present, but the latter is unusually not associated with an increased risk of atherosclerosis. Ursodeoxycholic acid (urso) has been shown in some studies to be an effective treatment, normalising liver function tests and delaying histological progression. It is generally accepted that urso treatment increases life expectancy. Colchicine and metho-trexate are also used in some centres but there is little conclusive evidence that immunosupressants (including prednisolone) are of use.

3.3   E: Start an *N*-acetylcysteine infusion

In any patient in whom a significant paracetamol overdose is suspected it is worth starting an *N*-acetylcysteine infusion pending further information and blood test results. If considered, gastric lavage should be done within 4 hours of ingestion. Hypoglycaemia may occur in fulminant liver failure. Transplant should be considered if the pH falls below 7.31, the prothrombin time exceeds 100 seconds or the creatinine exceeds 300 μmol/l. Psychiatric input is helpful in the management of any patient who has taken an intentional overdose, but should only be sought only once the patient is medically stable.

3.4   E: Pernicious anaemia

Pernicious anaemia and chronic pancreatitis may both contribute to vitamin B_{12} deficiency. The latter is unlikely in the absence of a history of alcohol excess or pain. Coeliac disease may present with anaemia and may be associated with neurological consequences through malabsorption. However, it would normally cause a normocytic or microcytic anaemia, as iron absorption is impaired as well as the absorption of folate, and to a much lesser extent than B_{12}. Body stores of B_{12} can last several years without replacement so the relatively short history of weight loss makes poor appetite a much less likely answer. Vitamin C can impair iron absorption.

3.5   D: The use of a non-selective β-blocker such as propranolol to maintain portal pressure below 12 mmHg

Oesophageal varices develop in portal hypertension as a consequence of porto-systemic shunting of blood through intrinsic and extrinsic gastro-oesophageal veins. Guidelines on the management of variceal haemorrhage were published by the British Society of Gastroenterologists in 2000. Around 30–50% of people with portal hypertension will have an episode of variceal bleeding and the mortality for a first bleed is as high as 50%. For this reason primary prophylaxis (ie the treatment of varices found at endoscopy that have never bled) is recommended. Physiological studies show that a reduction of the trans hepatic venous pressure gradient to below 12 mmHg prevents variceal bleeding and this has become the aim of prophylactic therapy. The mainstay of long-term prophylaxis is pharmacological with the most evidence for use of propranolol, a non-selective β-blocker, to reduce portal pressure by lowering cardiac output and causing splanchnic vasoconstriction. If β-blockers are not tolerated eradication of varices with serial endoscopic band ligation can be used but sclerotherapy has not been shown to be effective in this context. Vasopressin analogues only have a place in the treatment of acute variceal haemorrhage.

3.6   D: Serum Potassium monitoring is essential

NICE published guidelines on nutritional support in adults in 2006. These guidelines set the ideal total energy intake (including protein) at 25–35 kcal/kg per day for a patient in hospital. The guidelines highlight the dangers of refeeding syndrome in vulnerable individuals. Large nutritional loads in patients who have undergone a period of severe malnutrition can lead to life threatening electrolyte disturbances and for this reason it is recommended that at risk individuals be commenced on 5–10 kcal/kg per day.

The criteria for determining individuals at high risk of developing refeeding problems are one or more of the following:

- body mass index (BMI) less than 16 kg/m^2
- unintentional weight loss greater than 15% within the last few months
- little or no nutritional intake for more than 10 days
- low levels of potassium, phosphate or magnesium before feeding

or two or more of the following:

- BMI less than 18.5 kg/m^2
- unintentional weight loss greater than 10% within the last few months
- little or no nutritional intake for more than 5 days
- a history of alcohol abuse or drugs including insulin, chemotherapy, antacids and diuretics.

Patients at risk should be supplemented with high dose thiamine and vitamin B preparations as well as other micronutrients for at least the first 10 days of feeding and should have careful monitoring and replacement of serum electrolytes. The NICE guidelines also support the use of parenteral nutrition only in those patients in whom enteral feeding has failed or is impractical. In most cases nasogastric feeding will be the method of choice in severely ill patients.

3.7   E: Troublesome perianal Crohn's disease

HIV infection is often associated with past or present hepatitis B and C infection with which it shares common routes of transmission. Diarrhoea is a troublesome symptom for patients with HIV, sometimes associated with organisms such as *Cryptosporidium,* which normally pose no risk for immunocompetent individuals. Although a few case reports suggest that active Crohn's disease may co-exist with advanced HIV infection, more often the immunosuppression due to HIV suppresses Crohn's disease activity.

3.8   C: A single dose of ciprofloxacin may be of benefit

Travellers' diarrhoea is estimated to affect 20–50% of travellers from resource rich to resource poor countries. The commonest responsible organism is enterotoxic *Escherichia coli;* others include *Campylobacter, Salmonella* spp, *Shigella, Cryptosporidium, Giardia* and enteric viruses. Most infections are self-limiting and the mainstay of treatment is rehydration. Commercial rehydration salts are available but the WHO recommend a homemade solution of eight level teaspoons of sugar and $\frac{1}{2}$ teaspoon of salt in 1 litre of clean water. In travellers for whom symptoms would be inconvenient (businessmen, athletes, people undertaking long journeys by car or train etc) a single 500 mg dose of ciprofloxacin has been shown to be of benefit especially combined with loperamide.

Three per cent of travellers' diarrhoea lasts for longer than 1 month. Forty two per cent of reported cases of travel-associated diarrhoea reported in the UK is after trips to Europe (compared with 21% to Africa and the Middle East, 8% to South East Asia and the Far East and 1% to South America) mostly due to the higher frequency of travel to these countries, although it is a pertinent reminder that good food hygiene should be followed whatever the destination.

3.9   A: A low-alcohol lager

Only the beer contains a proscribed cereal, barley-derived hops.

3.10   C: She must be sent to hospital as she is dehydrated and pyrexial: given the history you are concerned to diagnose and treat any antibiotic-associated complications as soon as possible

Confusion, pyrexia, dehydration and diarrhoea are all symptoms and signs that may necessitate admission, if only for care, in an elderly person living alone at home – although not every elderly person with just one of these symptoms could be admitted! While metronidazole is the preferred treatment for *Clostridium difficile*-associated diarrhoea in the UK, it too may cause *C. difficile* overgrowth. Relapse after apparently successful treatment is not uncommon.

C. difficile is becoming an increasing problem in the UK with over 44 000 cases reported in 2005. Eighty per cent of cases occur in the over-65 age group. In the recent years the emergence of a new strain (Type027) has caused a number of serious outbreaks in North America, The Netherlands and the UK. Type027 produces 10–20 times the amount of toxin A and B, which are the elements responsible for the pathogenicity of the organism, and consequently mortality and morbidity rates are increased.

3.11   B: The persistent back ache is a poor prognostic sign

The British Society of Gastroenterology published guidelines on the management of pancreatic cancers in 2005. Pancreatic cancer is problematic as it presents late, often when curative resection is impossible. Average survival for patients with unresectable disease is 2–3 months. Risk factors for the development of pancreatic cancer include cigarette smoking, previous acute pancreatitis and a diagnosis of diabetes within the last 2 years. Poor prognostic clinical indicators including abdominal mass, persistent back pain, ascites, marked and rapid weight loss and supraclavicular lymphadenopathy are associated with unresectability.

Diagnosis is usually made using several radiographic modalities and endoscopic ultrasound provides a method of assessment and an avenue for tissue diagnosis. Transperitoneal biopsy has limited sensitivity in patients with potentially resectable tumours and should be avoided.

In unresectable tumours, palliative chemotherapy with gemcitabine has been shown to be of benefit in several large trials giving a modest survival benefit and symptom improvement. Coeliac plexus neurolysis can often be performed endoscopically and can provide excellent relief from back pain.

3.12   C: If she has had her small bowel resected she may be malabsorbing folic acid and so supplementation at a higher than normal dose would be advised

Folic acid supplements are recommended for all pregnant women as their need for folate rises five-fold. Folate is denatured through overcooking. Liver is contraindicated in pregnancy through concern about its high vitamin A content. Blind-loop bacteria tend to consume vitamin B_{12} and produce folate.

3.13   C: His family's description of an inversion of his normal sleep pattern

Hepatic encephalopathy is a complication of both acute and chronic liver disease and its exact pathogenesis remains elusive. It is likely to be in part due to increased ammonia levels in the brain, altered levels of neuronal amino acids and the presence of false neurotransmitters. Chronic hepatic encephalopathy can be difficult to detect but one of the earliest signs is reversal of sleep pattern; this can lean on to drowsiness or agitation and progress to coma and death. Reflexes are preserved and brisk reflexes and positive plantar signs are not uncommon. Although confusion does occur it is not a specific sign of hepatic encephalopathy. Headache again is a non-specific symptom, which is diagnostically unhelpful in this case.

3.14   D: Offer advice on laxatives

Solitary rectal ulcers are typically found on the anterior rectal wall in young women with a history of constipation, and may reflect strain-associated prolapse. While an uncommon cause of anaemia, in this case other more common causes appear to have been excluded. The histology will differentiate between inflammatory bowel disease and solitary rectal ulcer disease but, given the history, a trial of laxatives rather than mesalazine seems an appropriate next step pending biopsy results.

3.15   D: Coeliac serology should be checked

The British Society of Gastroenterologists published guidelines on the management of iron deficiency anaemia (IDA) in 2005. They recommend the upper and lower gastrointestinal (GI) investigation in all cases of confirmed IDA in men and postmenopausal women. IDA occurs in 5–12% of otherwise healthy premenopausal women and does not require GI investigations unless there are specific symptoms or strong family history of bowel cancer. Coeliac disease is responsible for approximately 4% of all cases of IDA in this group and therefore serological testing is advised.

Renal tract blood loss is responsible for 1% of all cases of IDA and therefore urine dipstick should be a routine part of investigation. It has been estimated that blood donation may be responsible for up to 5% of IDA.

3.16   E: He should be screened for anaemia

NICE guidelines for the management of adult dyspepsia in the community were published in 2004. Non-ulcer dyspepsia is common and does not require extensive investigation in all patients. First-line endoscopy is recommended only in patients with specific symptoms (gastrointestinal (GI) blood loss, iron deficiency anaemia, progressive/unintentional weight loss, dysphagia, persistent vomiting, epigastric mass or abnormal barium meal) or in patients over the age of 55 with new onset symptoms. Treatment options include simple lifestyle advice (such as weight reduction and smoking cessation), which may be effective in many cases, or trials of proton pump inhibitors (PPIs) or H_2 receptor antagonists. *Helicobacter pylori* may be responsible for some cases of non-ulcer dyspepsia but should only be treated after a positive breath, stool antigen or serological test. Retesting is not recommended. If symptoms persist the mainstay of therapy are antisecretory drugs (PPIs or H_2 receptor antagonists) but the aim should be to wean patients off drugs in the long term if possible.

3.17   D: He requires a liver biopsy

Wilson's disease is an autosomal recessive disease with a world-wide incidence estimated at 30/million population. The genetic defect results in abnormalities of a metal transporting P-type ATPase, which results in a decrease in copper excretion into the bile. The inability to transport copper within the hepatocyte results in reduced circulating levels of the copper transport protein ceruloplasmin.

Wilson's disease can manifest in several ways with mainly hepatic disease (ranging from mild abnormalities of liver function to cirrhosis or acute liver failure), neurological or psychiatric presentations.

The American Association for the Study of Liver Disease published guidelines on the diagnosis and management of Wilson's disease in 2003. The guidelines highlight the diagnostic difficulty in this disease, as no one test is definitive. A mildly low ceruloplasmin is not diagnostic (a very low test is more suggestive). Kayser–Fleischer rings are associated with 95% of cases with neurological presentations, but only 50–60% of patients with mainly hepatic disease. A liver biopsy with calculation of dry weight copper is felt to be the most reliable way to establish a diagnosis in adulthood. Although the defective gene has been identified it is very large and over 200 mutations have so far been identified. It is of use in family studies or in certain populations where a single mutation predominates (eg parts of Japan, Iceland and the Canary Islands).

The initial treatment of Wilson's disease is with chelating agents (eg penicillamine or trientine), which aid excretion of copper in the urine. Once copper levels have been lowered maintenance therapy with zinc salts (that interfere with copper absorption in the gut) can be started but lifelong pharmacological treatment for all established cases is necessary to prevent relapse.

3.18   C: He may have a genetic polymorphism on chromosome 2

The most likely cause of an isolated rise in bilirubin in an otherwise healthy individual is Gilbert's syndrome. This is an isolated unconjugated hyperbilirubinaemia present in an estimated 7–10% of the population and caused by impairment of hepatic conjugation pathways. The commonest defect is in bilirubin–uridine diphosphonate glucuronyl transferase (UGT), an enzyme product of the *UGT-1* gene on chromosome 2. Affected individuals have benign isolated rises in bilirubin associated with dehydration, fasting, intercurrent illness, trauma and intense exercise. Bilirubin levels rarely exceed 50 μmol/l and levels > 100 μmol/l should lead to further investigation for other causes. Some affected individuals seem to experience vague abdominal pain for which no other cause is found but in this case the symptoms are likely to be due to an intercurrent illness. Low-grade haemolytic anaemia can coexist with and exacerbate Gilbert's – haemolytic processes do not necessarily result in persistently low haemoglobins and can themselves be exacerbated by intercurrent illness.

3.19   A: Genetic testing may aid diagnosis

Haemochromatosis describes the clinical syndrome of iron overload while genetic haemochromatosis is a term generally reserved for iron overload resulting from mutations of the *HFE* gene on chromosome 6. In the UK, 90% of patients with genetic haemochromatosis are homozygous for the C282Y mutation with 4% being C282Y/H63D compound heterozygotes. Serum ferritin is often used as a screen for haemochromatosis, but it is an acute phase protein and can be elevated in acute illness and is also often high in alcohol related liver disease. A liver biopsy is useful to aid diagnosis; if there is evidence of liver dysfunction (abnormal liver function tests (LFTs) and suggestion of cirrhosis on ultrasound) the pattern of iron deposition within the liver as well as calculation of total iron content will enable differentiation between alcohol-related iron overload and genetic haemochromatosis. Normal total body iron content is 4–5 g with 3 g held within haemoglobin – in haemochromatosis total body iron could reach levels of up to 40 g. Venesection is the treatment of choice in haemochromatosis with 250 mg of iron removed with each 500 ml of blood. Its role in iron overload associated with alcohol-related liver disease is not established.

3.20   D: A C-reactive protein (CRP) > 150 mg/l at 48 hours is a poor prognostic indicator

The British Society of Gastroenterology published guidelines on the management of acute pancreatitis in 2005. Acute pancreatitis has an incidence of 150–420 cases/million population and clinically presents with abdominal pain, vomiting and a raised serum amylase. The guidelines state that a cause for pancreatitis should be found in at least 80% of cases (gallstone disease accounts for 50% and alcohol for 25%).

Plain abdominal films are unhelpful in diagnosis – abdominal ultrasound scan (USS) may show a swollen oedematous pancreas but pancreatic visualisation is possible in only 25–30% of cases. Computed tomography (CT) scans can visualise the pancreas, but the timing of examination is contentious and early diagnostic CT scan is not routinely performed in the UK.

Poor prognostic features that suggest the progression to complications (pancreatic necrosis) include clinical impression of severity, obesity (body mass index (BMI) > 30 kg/m^2), APACHE II score > 8 in the first 24 hours of admission and CRP > 150 mg/l, Glasgow score 30 or more or persistant organ failure at 48 hours.

The treatment of acute pancreatitis is supportive with specialist management, adequate and prompt fluid resuscitation and oxygen therapy identified as particularly crucial. The role of prophylactic antibiotics to prevent infection of necrotic pancreatic tissue is controversial with some trials showing benefit and others showing none. The guidelines state that there is still not enough evidence to definitively support the use of prophylactic antibiotics in acute pancreatitis.

3.21   B: You arrange upper gastrointestinal (GI) tract endoscopy

Dysphagia (difficulty in swallowing) and odynophagia (painful swallowing) together require investigation unless they settle rapidly with empirical measures. Trials show that a negative endoscopy may in itself help the patient's symptoms to settle. Endoscopy is usually done as a precursor to oesophageal physiology studies, though barium fluoroscopy may provide information on both structure and motility. Psychological support may be helpful in the management of functional GI disturbance.

3.22   C: General anaesthesia should be avoided if possible

The UK Neuroendocrine Tumour Network published guidelines on the management of gastroenteropancreatic neuroendocrine tumours (NETs) in 2005. NETs represent a heterogeneous group of tumours that arise from neuroendocrine cells in the gastrointestinal (GI) tract, pancreas and bronchus. Many are secretory and associated with hypersecretory syndromes. Carcinoid tumours are a subset of NETs that once metastasised to the liver produce the carcinoid syndrome (characterised by flushing and diarrhoea), due to the release of serotonin and other vasoactive substances into the general circulation. Carcinoid crisis is a life-threatening condition characterised by profound flushing, bronchospasm, tachycardia and fluctuating blood pressure. It can occur in patients with carcinoid tumours during the induction of any general anaesthesia, or the handling or destruction of the tumours during treatment. The crisis can be prevented by pretreatment with octreotide infusions.

Diagnosis is made by histology, radiology (including computed tomography (CT) and magnetic resonance imaging (MRI)). Labelled octreotide scans are useful for detecting metastasis as NETs preferentially express somatostatin receptors (which bind octreotide). Carcinoid tumours were traditionally diagnosed using 24-hour urinary 5-hydroxyindole acetic acid (5-HIAA) levels but these can be negative in foregut carcinoid tumours. Chromogranin A is a protein of unknown function that is secreted by the majority of neuroendocrine tumours and is therefore a more sensitive marker.

Some neuroendocrine tumours are associated with type 1 multiple endocrine neoplasia syndromes (MEN1), particularly insulinomas and gastrinomas. Gut carcinoids are not associated with this condition although the guidelines recommend that anyone diagnosed with any NET be screened for MEN1 and MEN2.

3.23   E: Maintenance therapy may reduce the risk of colon cancer

Guidelines on the management of ulcerative colitis were published in 2004 by the British Society of Gastroenterology. Recommendations for first-line maintenance therapy are the newer 5-ASA drugs (mesalazine or balsalazide) as they have fewer side-effects than the parent drug sulfasalazine. Azathioprine has been shown to be effective in the maintenance of remission in ulcerative colitis, but its toxicity profile means that its use should be reserved for patients with frequent relapses on other drugs. There is no good evidence to support the long-term use of steroids in the maintenance of either ulcerative colitis or Crohn's disease. The use of 5-ASA compounds has been shown to reduce the risk of colon cancer by up to 75%, supporting its long-term use in extensive ulcerative colitis, but in mild distal disease that has been in remission for several years discontinuing all therapy is an option that should be discussed with the patient.

3.24   C: Acarbose might be of use in symptomatic control

This woman's symptoms are typical of postgastrectomy dumping syndrome. Dumping syndromes can be early (occurring within 60 minutes of eating) or late (1–3 hours postprandially). Both types are caused by rapid transit of osmotically active solids and liquids into the small bowel. In early dumping, fluids are drawn into the large bowel and cause bloating and abdominal pain – increases in gut hormone release are also thought to be a component. In late dumping delivery of large amounts of carbohydrates to the proximal small bowel and consequent massive glucose absorption cause an exaggerated insulin response leading to symptoms of hypoglycaemia.

An insulinoma in the stomach would be highly unlikely and would not resemble a gastrointestinal stromal tumour (GIST) histologically. The malignant potential of GISTs is accurately classified according to size and numbers of mitotic figures – recurrence of a very low risk tumour would be very unusual.

Acarbose prevents glucose absorption and along with octreotide is effective for symptom relief in dumping syndrome. Prokinetic agents would exacerbate the problems in this case.

3.25 E: Symptoms of vomiting within 4 hours and diarrhoea within 10 hours suggest *Bacillus cereus* as a likely cause

E. histolytica tends to cause a sudden onset of bloody diarrhoea 12–24 hours after ingestion. *Campylobacter* species are most commonly found in contaminated animal products. Canned foods classically harbour *Clostridium botulinum* toxin. *Vibrio parahaemolyticus* is found in seafood. Enterotoxic *Escherichia coli* can affect young and old, fit and disabled alike, although is more likely to be life threatening in the very young or frail elderly.

3.26 E: Primary sclerosing cholangitis

The cholestatic picture in conjunction with the ulcerative colitis history and positive antineutrophil cytoplasmic antibody (ANCA) would favour a diagnosis of primary sclerosing cholangitis (PSC). PSC is a cholangiopathy of uncertain (probably autoimmune) aetiology. It occurs in 3–10% of ulcerative colitis patients and should be suspected if the alkaline phosphatase is unexpectedly raised (jaundice is a late sign). Progressive cholestasis and cholangitis lead to death unless cure is achieved with liver transplantation. There is a 10–30% incidence of cholangiocarcinoma in PSC.

Viral hepatitis would be expected to cause a significant rise in alanine aminotransferase (ALT) and jaundice. Incidental common bile duct damage can occur at the time of surgery but usually results in structuring and dilatation which would be evident on ultrasound. Primary biliary cirrhosis is unlikely in a man in this age group. Metachronous colorectal metastasis from bowel cancer is an unlikely possibility as colons removed electively for ulcerative colitis are examined for the presence of incidental malignancy.

3.27 C: Bacterial overgrowth secondary to an enterocolic fistula

This is a picture of malabsorption for which the main differential diagnoses are active small bowel Crohn's disease and a fistula, with bacterial overgrowth. The laboratory tests do not indicate an inflammatory process. Acquired lactose intolerance can give bloating and diarrhoea, but not anaemia or low albumin. Bile salt diarrhoea is watery, but not associated with colic or systemic symptoms. Strictures are associated with colic, but will not cause anaemia and a low albumin unless there is bacteria overgrowth too. So, only a fistula with overgrowth will fully explain the symptoms.

3.28   A: Coeliac disease

This is a picture of malabsorption. 'Silent' malabsorption of this type strongly suggests coeliac disease. The mouth ulcers are associated with coeliac disease or Crohn's disease, but there are no other symptoms to suggest Crohn's disease. In general, giardiasis and Crohn's disease are associated with gastrointestinal symptoms in addition to malabsorption. Scleroderma has characteristic extra-intestinal signs.

3.29   B: Treatment with Glivec may be necessary

Gastrointestinal stromal tumours (GISTs) are soft tissue sarcomas arising from mesenchymal cells in the gastrointestinal (GI) tract and encompass tumours previously classified as leiomyomas and leiomyosarcomas. GISTs have an estimated incidence of 15/million population and account for 0.1–3% of all gastrointestinal (GI) cancers. A total of 60–70% occur in the stomach and abdominal pain and GI bleeding are common presentations.

All GISTs are considered to have a malignant potential although the risk can be stratified according to tumour size and numbers of mitotic figures seen in the tumour. Tumours less than 2 cm in diameter have a very low malignant potential and may be left in situ and observed for size increase. Percutaneous biopsy is not advised due to the risk of malignant seeding and surgical removal without a tissue diagnosis is usually advocated. The treatment for GIST is surgical resection including en bloc dissection of adjacent involved structures.

GISTs all express the tyrosine kinase KIT (CD117) and this has been the target of therapy for unresectable or metastasised tumours. Imatinib (Glivec) was developed as a selective inhibitor of KIT and its use leads to tumour stability in many patients. It is highly selective and does not inhibit other tyrosine kinases required for normal cell function and therefore has an acceptable side-effect profile.

3.30   A: Barium enema

Occult blood loss in a man of this age is due to a caecal cancer until proved otherwise. This is the age at which the incidence of such cancers rises significantly. Faecal occult blood (FOB) testing is pointless and, in the absence of overt blood loss, a non-vegetarian either has malabsorption or gastrointestinal (GI) bleeding; a negative FOB would not rule out bleeding. A red cell scan is only useful during an episode of bleeding. Upper GI malignancy is less common, but should be sought if the barium enema is normal.

3.31   C: Reassure her with explanation of the diagnosis, without further investigation

Her symptoms are those of irritable bowel syndrome. In most patients the cause is stress. Investigations are not called for in patients of this age, if at any age. Reassurance with a careful explanation of the problem is all that is usually required.

3.32   C: Budesonide could be used to maintain remission once induced

Guidelines on the management of Crohn's disease were published in 2006 by the European Crohn's and Colitis Organisation. These guidelines state that the diagnosis of mild exacerbations of Crohn's is difficult and that alternative explanations for symptoms should be sought. In mild disease studies have shown that up to 20% of patients will enter remission with placebo treatment and therefore no active treatment is an option if this is undertaken with the patient's support. Treatment of disease depends on activity and the site of the disease. Meta-analysis of the use of 5-ASA compounds in mild ileo-caecal disease has shown them to be only marginally better than placebo and less effective than oral budesonide. Budesonide is considered to be preferable to prednisolone because although it is marginally less effective its use does not lead to steroid associated side-effects.

Neither 5-ASA nor prednisolone has been shown to be effective in the maintenance of remission of ileo-caecal Crohn's. Budesonide has been shown to delay relapse for up to 12 months. Azathioprine is the most effective drug for long-term maintenance. Although elemental diets are used as therapy for Crohn's disease in children they are unpalatable and difficult to administer in adults and are not a useful alternative treatment in this situation.

3.33   D: High-dose proton pump inhibitor (PPI), reducing later

NICE guidelines support the stance of most gastroenterologists – to use an effective PPI, the dose of which is reduced once symptoms come under control. In patients of this age, who are unlikely to be taking other drugs and so are not at risk of drug interactions, price is the main determinant of the choice of PPI. A cost–effectiveness study has shown that antireflux surgery is not useful in most patients as they relapse later and then need to take PPI therapy once more.

3.34   D: Paracentesis/albumin/glypressin

This is type 1 hepatorenal failure. It occurs in patients with cirrhosis complicated by ascites and mild stable renal impairment (type 2 hepatorenal syndrome) who then have reduced renal perfusion due to sepsis or blood loss. The untreated mortality is 90% at 2 weeks, but the paracentesis/albumin/glypressin regimen lowers mortality and corrects renal failure in most patients.

3.35   B: Hepatitis A

This woman shows signs of fulminant hepatic failure with hepatic encephalopathy jaundice and prolonged clotting (as evidenced by the bleeding venipuncture site). In this situation, urgent referral to a transplant centre is required and liver transplantation is life saving. The most likely cause in view of the history is of hepatitis A, which can be contracted from seafood taken from sewage-contaminated seawater in endemic areas. Aspirin overdose does not cause liver failure. Hepatitis C is very rarely fulminant and there are no obvious risk factors for inoculation. Paracetamol overdose is a possibility and should be excluded with serum paracetamol measurements even in the face of strong denial from close relatives, as it is potentially treatable.

3.36   D: Primary biliary cirrhosis

Primary biliary cirrhosis is the most likely diagnosis. Itching can often be the first symptom and can occur before liver function derangement. It can be hard to treat and drugs such as ursodeoxycholic acid, colestyramine, rifampicin and naloxone have all been trialed with mixed success. Recent reports of the use of albumin dialysis (MARS therapy) to treat itching have been favourable and transplantation has been used for patients whose lives are blighted by intractable itching. The presence of antimitochondrial antibodies would confirm the diagnosis.

3.37   A: He is more likely to die of liver disease than AIDS

The common routes of transmission of HIV hepatitis B and C mean that co-infection with two or more of these viruses is common. It is estimated that 40% of patients with HIV also have hepatitis C. With the advent of improved combination antiretroviral drugs HIV has become a chronic disease, but liver damage secondary to viral hepatitis is accelerated and in the west it has become the biggest cause of mortality in the co-infected population.

For this reason all patients with HIV should be counselled about reducing risk and offered vaccination against hepatitis B – this is likely to be successful unless there is severe immunodeficiency. The treatment of hepatitis C remains the same as in the monoinfected population although the response rate to therapy may be slightly lower. In end-stage hepatitis C liver transplantation remains an option and stable HIV disease is no longer considered an absolute contraindication to this procedure. Hepatitis B and C do not affect the course of HIV disease but some antiretroviral agents (eg didanosine and stavudine) are contraindicated in liver disease due to the risk of lactic acidosis and liver decompensation.

3.38   C: Oesophageal variceal endoscopic ligation

British Society of Gastroenterology guidelines on the management of acute variceal haemorrhage were published in 2000. The guidelines recommend endoscopic evaluation and band ligation as the treatment of choice for bleeding oesophageal varices. If endoscopy is not available vasopressin analogues such as glypressin are useful and if bleeding continues balloon tamponade with a Sengstaken–Blakemore tube is indicated. Transjugular intrahepatic portosystemic shunt (TIPS) placement decompresses the portal system and allows access to large varices to enable embolisation. It is useful in patients who continue to bleed after endoscopic therapy, particularly if gastric varices are present. Intravenous propranolol has no place in the management of acute variceal bleeding as the reduction in cardiac output exacerbates hypotension from hypovolaemia and could be life threatening.

3.39   A: Azathioprine

Azathioprine is the only option to consider at this stage. Long-term steroids are not indicated in Crohn's disease. Ciclosporin does not work. Infliximab is only licensed for active disease that is refractory to steroids and first-line immuno-suppressives. Methotrexate causes miscarriage.

3.40   E: Serum ascites–albumin gradient (SAAG) is likely to be ≥ 11 g/l

The British Society of Gastroenterology have published guidelines on the management of ascites in 2006. Spontaneous bacterial peritonitis (SBP) occurs in around 15% of patients admitted to hospital with ascites and patients may have little in the way of clinical signs. All individuals admitted with ascites should therefore have a diagnostic ascitic tap (10–15 ml of fluid) and fluid sent for microscopy and culture. A neutrophil count of > 250 indicates spontaneous bacterial peritonitis (SBP). Two per cent of patients will have a bloody tap and in 50% of these no cause will be found, and 30% will have hepatocellular carcinoma as an underlying diagnosis.

Placing fluid into sterile containers for transport to a microbiology laboratory for subsequent culture will identify a causative organism in 40% of cases of SBP. This yield can be increased to around 80% by inoculating fluid into blood culture bottle at the bedside. Analysing total protein content of the ascitic fluid and classifying it as a transudate or exudate is unhelpful as up to 30% of patients with uncomplicated ascites will have ascitic fluid protein > 25 g/l. The serum ascites–albumin gradient is more useful (calculated by subtracting the ascitic albumin concentration from the serum albumin concentration) and is accurate in 97% of cases. An SAAG value of ⩾ 11 g/l indicates cirrhosis, nephritic syndrome or cardiac failure as a cause of ascites while a value of < 11 g/l indicates malignancy, pancreatitis or tuberculosis as possible causes.

The management of ascites includes the use of diuretics, large volume paracentesis and sodium restriction. Currently it is recommended that patients adopt a 'no added salt' diet (no salt added to food during cooking or at the table); this reduces daily sodium intake to 90 mmol/l. More severe sodium restrictions were used in the past but make the diet unpalatable and lead to malnutrition. Bed rest has not been shown to be of benefit and should not be encouraged as it increases co-morbidity.

3.41   D: Proton pump inhibitor (PPI) treatment with repeat endoscopy in 3 to 6 months

There is a significant risk of Barrett's oesophagus and adenocarcinoma arising in such a patient. Peptic strictures may also occur. Severe oesophagitis may lead to dysphagia even without a stricture. Severe dysplasia should be confirmed by repeat endoscopy in the presence of acid blockade. If confirmed, oesophagectomy should be performed.

3.42   E: Solitary rectal ulcer

The site of the lesion is characteristic. Solitary rectal ulcers are associated with straining at stool and trauma (due to digitally assisted evacuation for example). The lesion may resemble a tumour, so a biopsy is essential.

3.43   C: Pneumatosis coli

The gas-filled blebs are characteristic. Pneumatosis coli is associated with chronic obstructive pulmonary disease (COPD) and usually presents with rectal bleeding and diarrhoea. Antibiotic diarrhoea may be accompanied by blood and is a reasonable thought in a patient likely to have been exposed to antibiotics, but the duration of the symptoms is too long. The patient is too old to have familial adenomatous polyposis.

3.44   A: Cytomegalovirus (CMV) proctitis

Cytomegalovirus (CMV) proctitis is painless, unlike herpes proctitis. Inclusion bodies are characteristic.

3.45   D: Portal vein thrombosis

Bleeding oesophageal varices in the absence of signs of chronic liver disease strongly suggest portal vein thrombosis. Special Care Baby Unit (SCBU) treatment is likely to be associated with umbilical vein cannulation with the attendant risk of sepsis and portal vein thrombosis.

3.46   B: Hydatid disease

Hydatid disease is usually asymptomatic. The infestation is acquired by exposure to faeces containing *Echinococcus* eggs. The internal acoustic shadows are the key to the ultrasonographic diagnosis.

3.47   E: It stimulates pancreatic exocrine secretion

Cholecystokinin is related to secretin. Its actions include causing the gallbladder to contract and stimulating pancreatic production of lipases in response to a fatty meal. While it does delay gastric emptying it does so via a vagal reflex rather than direct action on the muscularis.

3.48   E: Peristomal abscess

Peristomal inflammation will lead to diarrhoea. The investigations are consistent with an abscess. Bile salt diarrhoea only occurs if the colon is in continuity. *Clostridium* is pathogenic only in the large bowel.

3.49   E: He will be at increased risk of renal calculi

Crohn's disease is one of the commonest causes of short bowel syndrome. Guidelines for the management of patients with a short bowel were published by the British Society of Gastroenterology in 2006. Normal human small intestine length (measured from the duodenojejunal flexure) can range from 275 cm to 850 cm and therefore it is the length of small bowel *remaining* that is important in determining likely sequelae. The problems associated with small bowel are variable but in general patients with an intact colon are unlikely to require long-term enteral or parenteral nutrition as the colon takes over absorptive function.

Patients with jejunostomies are more likely to require nutritional and fluid support as stomal loses can be high. The restriction of enteral fluid intake can help reduce stoma output and electrolyte loss. Hypomagnesaemia occurs because of chelation of magnesium by non-absorbed fatty acids and increased renal excretion (because of secondary hyperaldosteronism).

Patients with a jejuno-colic anastomosis have a 25% chance of developing symptomatic calcium oxalate renal stones due to increased oxalate absorption in the colon – they should be advised to remain on a low oxalate diet.

3.50   A: Boerhaave's syndrome

This is a characteristic presentation of this life-threatening disorder. The oesophagus is ruptured during severe vomiting. Perforation usually occurs to the left, giving rise to mediastinal and pericardial emphysema and a left pleural effusion.

ANSWERS

Nephrology

4.1   A: Fluid entering the distal tubule is hypo-osmolar

In the descending limb of the loop of Henle, water is passively reabsorbed through aquaporin channels. The ascending limb lacks aquaporin channels. Active excretion of Na from the water-impermeable ascending limb creates hypo-osmolar urine as it enters the collecting duct. Pumping of NaCl from the ascending limb to the descending limb creates a hyper-osmotic medullary interstitium around the tip of the loop of Henle. When the collecting duct travels through this medium, water travels out of the lumen (via antidiuretic hormone (ADH)-dependent aquaporin channels) to concentrate the urine. ANP causes a diuresis by increasing glomerular filtration. This results in a less hyper-osmolar medullary interstium, and hence less water re-absorption. Thiazides act on the Na-Cl co-transporters in the distal tubule. Amiloride is active at the Na channel in the collecting duct.

4.2   A: Diffuse proliferative glomerulonephritis

The clinical scenario should point you to lupus nephritis, which is by far the most likely unifying diagnosis. You then need to recall the five most common renal histological appearances of lupus nephritis:

- normal
- mesangial deposits/hypercellularity
- focal segmental proliferative glomerulonephritis
- diffuse proliferative glomerulonephritis
- membranous glomerulonephritis.

Pauci-immune focal necrotising glomerulonephritis is rarely seen in lupus, and is far more commonly associated with Wegener's disease. There is nothing in this clinical scenario to suggest a diagnosis of cholesterol embolisation, interstitial nephritis, or amyloidosis (characterised histologically by Congo red staining).

4.3   D: MRA of renal arteries

Biopsy of the small kidney would be technically difficult and reveal no useful information. Biopsy of the large kidney would effectively carry the same risk as biopsy of a single kidney, which is carried out very rarely. IVP will not be useful, as the dye will not concentrate adequately in this degree of renal failure. In addition it is potentially nephrotoxic.

In any case, there is a high clinical suspicion of renal artery disease, which is further augmented by the radiological finding of renal asymmetry. (The other main cause of renal asymmetry, chronic pyelonephritis, is much less likely in this clinical setting, and ultrasound would be likely to reveal cortical scarring in addition.)

Therefore the investigation of choice narrows to angiography and magnetic resonance angiogram (MRA). Because of its invasive nature and the risk of nephrotoxicity, angiography should generally be preceded by MRA.

4.4   B: Needle track marks

Facial oedema, thrombo-embolic disease, and hypertension may all be found in nephrotic syndrome and are not diagnostically useful. Unilateral ptosis in a woman of this age is likely to be congenital ptosis (ask her!). Horner's syndrome, in conjunction with an apical lung tumour and associated membranous glomerulonephritis is an unlikely possibility. Intravenous drug abusers are at risk of hepatitis B, C and HIV. Nephrotic syndrome is a possibility through membranous glomerulonephritis (hepatitis B) mesangiocapillary glomerulonephritis (hepatitis B or C) or HIV nephropathy (focal segmental glomerulosclerosis).

4.5   B: Nephrocalcinosis is rare

Renal tubular acidosis is a subject with which many candidates struggle. The best advice is probably not to spend fruitless hours trying to understand it, but for the purposes of the exam, to learn it. The following table may help.

	Distal (type I)	Proximal (type II)
Hypokalaemia	Severe	Moderate
HCO_3^- loss in urine	Small	Large
Response to HCO_3^- therapy	Good	Large doses required
Urine pH	Never less than 5.5	May acidify urine well if serum HCO_3^- low
Glycosuria, aminoaciduria, Fanconi's syndrome	No	Common
Nephrolithiasis, nephrocalcinosis, bone disease	Common	Not typical
Defect	Tubular secretion of H^+	HCO_3^- reabsorption

Type IV renal tubular acidosis is quite different, and is characterised by hyperkalaemic, hyperchloraemic acidosis, and reduced ammonium secretion. It is caused by mineralocorticoid insufficiency or by decreased end-organ response to aldosterone.

4.6   C: If the renal ultrasound shows large kidneys the condition may be chronic

Although renal anaemia generally develops gradually, there are a number of conditions (one thinks particularly of the haemolytic uraemic syndrome) in which substantial anaemia may occur in acute renal failure. Similarly, the degree of proteinuria is far more dependent on the underlying diagnosis than on the chronicity of the condition. Phosphate levels rise quickly in renal failure and are not necessarily indicative of chronic disease.

Although most causes of renal failure eventually end with renal atrophy, in certain conditions, most notably polycystic kidney disease, they will be enlarged. Cortical depth is a more useful indication, but may be hard to assess in polycystic disease. (However, the renal failure of polycystic disease is generally chronic in nature.) The acute nephritides will tend to show bright kidneys on ultrasound, the brightness becoming more marked with progression of the disease. At or near end-stage renal failure, the small bright kidneys are often indistinguishable from surrounding fat.

4.7   B: Anti-GBM assay

All of the following diagnoses are possible causes of crescentic nephritis: poststreptococcal glomerulonephritis; Goodpasture's syndrome; lupus; vasculitis; endocarditis. However, the causes of pulmonary–renal syndrome are somewhat different, Wegener's and Goodpasture's being at the top of the list, and most likely on this clinical history. The biopsy appearance is typical of Goodpasture's syndrome, where antibodies are deposited in a linear appearance along the glomerular basement membrane. In Wegener's, there is very little antibody deposition (pauci-immune crescentic nephritis), and in the other diagnoses suggested above, the immunofluorescence would tend to be granular.

What are we to make of the positive antineutrophil cytoplasmic antibody (ANCA) test? Firstly, it is important to remember the possibility of false positive testing with indirect immunofluorescence. We would wish to proceed to ELISA to confirm the diagnosis. However, the ELISA test we would expect to be positive in Wegener's (c-ANCA positive disease) is PR3 not MPO. The most likely diagnosis here is the Goodpasture's–Wegener's overlap syndrome, but you do not need to know that to answer this question correctly.

4.8 E: Alfacalcidol alone

There is no indication for a bisphosphonate in this patient with secondary hyperparathyroidism (renal osteodystrophy). There is likewise no indication for parathyroidectomy, which is reserved for patients with tertiary hyperparathyroidism, ie where the parathyroid hormone (PTH) level is (inappropriately) high despite elevated calcium levels. The therapeutic priority in this patient is to elevate the calcium towards the upper end of the normal range, which will help to suppress PTH activity. This is achieved by the prescription of alfacalcidol. However, alfacalcidol will also elevate the phosphate levels, and it is often necessary to prescribe a phosphate binder beforehand. This patient is already on sevelamer, an effective phosphate binder, and the serum phosphate levels are currently acceptable. The phosphate (and calcium) levels will need to be carefully monitored, but at present there is no indication to adjust his phosphate binders. In any case, phosphate binders (sevelamer, calcichew) must be given immediately before food to be effective.

4.9 D: Ramipril causes a preferential dilatation of the efferent glomerular arteriole resulting in a critical fall in glomerular filtration pressure

This should be a straightforward question, and the best way to approach it is probably to work out the correct answer before you look at the choices offered. Most of the others are frank nonsense, but in the tension of the exam, it is easy to be blinded by pseudoscience! Ramipril is not a medication typically associated with interstitial nephritis, and it certainly would not be the most likely explanation in this instance. Ramipril does reduce the conversion of angiotensin I to angiotensin II, but the mechanism of causing acute renal failure in patients with renal artery stenosis is more specific than its simple hypotensive effect (as described in option D). Ramipril has no direct effect on the action of aldosterone, nor on the juxtaglomerular apparatus.

4.10 C: Haemolytic uraemic syndrome (HUS)

This is a slightly tricky question, because the first three offered diagnoses (disseminated intravascular coagulation (DIC), thrombotic thrombocytopenic purpura (TTP) and HUS) are all part of a spectrum of disease, with sometimes unclear boundaries between them. First consider the other two possibilities. There is no such thing as 'delayed onset pre-eclampsia' in this context. While eclampsia may and does occasionally occur in a previously normotensive woman immediately after delivery, development of hypertension at 3 weeks post partum cannot possibly be pre-eclampsia. There is no evidence for toxic shock syndrome. In particular, the fact that she is severely hypertensive rules this out. The absence of skin bruising and a normal clotting profile should steer you away from a diagnosis of DIC.

This woman has post-partum HUS. It is a well-recognised entity, and the case described is typical. The normal clotting profile and absence of purpurae should not dissuade you from making this diagnosis. The clotting is typically normal in HUS, and while purpurae are commonly seen in the diarrhoeal form of the illness, they are a less common feature of the non-diarrhoeal forms. Confusion, however, tends to be more marked in these types. Renal biopsy, if performed would show a more severe pre-glomerular pathology than would be expected with the diarrhoeal forms of the disease. Intimal proliferation and obliteration is typical. Because of this, the renal prognosis will be somewhat guarded. The non-diarrhoeal forms of the illness are far more likely to result in chronic renal failure.

4.11 E: Focal segmental glomerulosclerosis

Clinically significant recurrence is particularly seen in focal segmental glomerulosclerosis (10–20%) and mesangiocapillary glomerulonephritis (around 15%). Membranous glomerulonephritis, IgA disease, and anti-GBM disease are often detected histologically, but it is rarely of major clinical significance. Lupus activity often subsides in end-stage renal failure and after transplantation. Scleroderma does not recur in the transplanted kidney. Diabetes may recur histologically, but the clinical manifestations are generally benign.

4.12 C: Chronic lumbar spine pain

This IVP appearance is typical of analgesic nephropathy. Therefore the history of longstanding back pain is highly relevant. Falciparum malaria may cause acute renal failure. On biopsy there is considerable tubular damage with relative glomerular sparing. The thalassaemia answer is intended to confuse you with sickle cell disease, which is a cause of papillary necrosis and similar IVP appearances to those described above. Hydrocarbons have been aetiologically implicated in Goodpasture's syndrome and Balkan nephropathy. Liquorice contains a mineralocorticoid-like substance; excess consumption can cause metabolic alkalosis and hypokalaemia.

4.13 A: Chronic obstructive pulmonary disease

Many patients who are completely blind are able to manage peritoneal dialysis very successfully. Diabetics do not have a strong requirement for either type of dialysis, although some find that the gentler fluid shifts of peritoneal dialysis (PD) are beneficial. For the same reason, patients with cardiovascular disease are likely to find PD an easier option. The rapid intravascular volume changes of haemodialysis present a significant stress to the cardiovascular system. Patients who are unable to adhere to fluid restrictions and who consistently attend the dialysis unit 4 or 5 kg over their 'dry weight' are likely to experience unpleasant side-effects from haemodialysis, especially cramps. They may in fact be unable to tolerate removal of all the fluid necessary, resulting in them coming off dialysis 'heavy', and perpetuating the problem for next time. Such patients are often more easily managed with the gentler fluid removal of PD. The fluid of peritoneal dialysis has a splinting effect on the diaphragm. For patients who already have respiratory compromise, this may cause significant respiratory embarrassment. Chronic obstructive pulmonary disease (COPD) is therefore quite a strong contraindication for peritoneal dialysis.

4.14   C: Lithium

When taken in excessive quantities, many drugs can cause acute renal failure even if this is not the primary symptom. The mechanism is commonly acute tubular necrosis, which may also occur following severe volume depletion. Haemodialysis is poor at removing drugs that have a large volume of distribution (eg amiodarone and paraquat) or are highly protein bound (eg digoxin and phenytoin). Haemodialysis may still be required to correct metabolic and fluid balance abnormalities that have occurred as a result of the renal failure.

4.15   D: Non-oliguria carries a better prognosis for long-term renal function than oliguria

Dopamine is used in low-doses to improve renal blood flow but this does not always lead to a diuresis. It is vital to ensure that a patient with renal failure is adequately hydrated before an attempt to stimulate a diuresis. Polyuria may occur in the recovery phase of acute tubular necrosis or as a result of nephrogenic diabetes insipidus, which may itself occur as a result of intermittent or partial obstruction. In all causes of renal failure non-oliguria carries a better prognosis than oliguria. Low plasma sodium almost always implies an excess of body water rather than a true deficit of body sodium; it gives no clue to tubular function. Hyaline casts are very non-specific, and are seen in health, after strenuous exercise, or in various renal conditions.

4.16   A: Chronic renal failure

In chronic renal failure, nocturia is often an early symptom. This increase of water excretion occurs because of the osmotic diuretic effect of raised urea and increasing insensitivity of the collecting tubules to antidiuretic hormone

(ADH). Acquired nephrogenic diabetes insipidus is associated with diseases that mainly affect the renal medulla. Hypokalaemic interstitial nephritis and the recovery phase of acute tubular necrosis (ATN) are examples of such diseases. However, hypokalaemia and hyperkalaemia themselves are not commonly associated with increased renal water excretion. Secondary hyper-aldosteronism occurs in hepatic and cardiac failure; this state is usually associated with volume overload, which occurs in association with a high renin level.

4.17   D: Urate 0.7 mmol/l

In the second and third trimesters of pregnancy glomerular filtration rate (GFR) increases and this is reflected by a decrease in both urea and creatinine. The serum concentrations of minerals such as magnesium are also characteristically low as a reflection of this. A rising uric acid level is a cause for concern as it is a possible indicator of the onset of pre-eclampsia.

4.18   E: Increase in venous volume

Renal sympathetic activity causes an increase in sodium reabsorption and a decrease in urinary sodium excretion. Similarly, a small fall in renal arterial pressure leads to an increase in proximal tubule reabsorption and decreased urinary excretion of sodium. An increase in venous volume leads to baroreceptor (atrial and renal capillary) signals, leading to increased sodium excretion. Increased plasma osmotic pressure increases proximal sodium reabsorption. All these mechanisms are involved in the maintenance of blood volume. Afferent and efferent arteriolar constriction is involved in autoregulation, maintaining glomerular filtration rate (GFR) and renal blood flow within narrow limits.

4.19   B: Compensation predominantly occurring at the proximal tubule

The renal response to this respiratory alkalosis is compensatory, restoring the pH to normal by metabolic compensation. The response is compensation rather than correction as the fall in the arterial partial pressure of carbon dioxide is not corrected; $p(CO_2)$ remains low. There is a decrease in the reabsorption of bicarbonate ions, which occurs mainly at the proximal tubule. This leads to a further fall in plasma bicarbonate and the pH will fall towards normal. Volume regulation is not a major part of the renal compensatory mechanisms of acid–base disturbances.

4.20   E: Renal sympathetic nervous stimulation causes increased renin release

Renin is a proteolytic enzyme released from the granular cells of the juxtaglomerular apparatus in response to sodium depletion (detected by cells of the macula densa) or volume depletion (detected by atrial and renal capillary baroreceptors). Reduced atrial stretch leads to increased renal sympathetic tone and renin release. Renin acts on angiotensinogen (renal substrate) to produce angiotensin I (later converted to angiotensin II, a potent vasoconstrictor). Angiotensin also stimulates thirst. Redistribution of blood away from the outer renal cortex stimulates renin release, which may be relevant to sodium retention in some disease states.

4.21   C: He takes atenolol for hypertension

Haemolytic disease of the newborn is the result of incompatibility of red cell antigens between mother and fetus; there is no association with uraemia occurring in later life. Drug history is an important part of the history in a patient with renal problems; in this scenario chronic analgesic usage and use of atenolol for hypertension are important factors. In addition to β-blockers, methysergide (a constituent of migraine therapies) may cause retroperitoneal fibrosis, a cause of renal failure. Childhood haematuria may indicate a progressive glomerulonephritis or a familial renal disease such as Alport's syndrome. Chronic exposure to silica, in foundry workers, can lead to heavy metal-type interstitial nephritis or glomerulosclerosis.

4.22   E: Retroperitoneal fibrosis by medial ureteric displacement on intravenous urograms

Renal obstruction is diagnosed by ultrasound; pressure studies may be required if the collecting system is dilated. Dehydration is itself a contraindication to performing intravenous urograms due to the increased risk of contrast nephropathy, particularly in diabetics, the elderly and arteriopaths; urograms will not aid diagnosis of dehydration. Coarse kidney scarring is caused by obstructive uropathy, papillary necrosis and renovascular disease in addition to reflux nephropathy. The diagnosis of retroperitoneal fibrosis is made by intravenous urograms; confirmation is made by biopsy of the peri-aortic mass seen on computed tomography (CT) or magnetic resonance imaging (MRI). Associations with retroperitoneal fibrosis include drugs (β-blockers, methyldopa, bromocriptine and methysergide) and carcinoid tumours. Large kidneys may indicate amyloidosis, diabetes or polycystic kidneys, so do not exclude parenchymal pathology.

4.23   E: Gold therapy for rheumatoid arthritis

Membranous glomerulonephritis accounts for 20–30% of adult nephrotic syndrome. It is associated with malignancy, autoimmune diseases and infections. It may be caused by a number of medications, including gold, penicillamine, captopril and NSAIDs. On renal biopsy the common findings are thickened basement membrane with IgG and C3 subepithelial deposition. End-stage renal failure occurs in approximately one-third of patients but usually over a period of several years from diagnosis. Highly selective proteinuria is more likely in minimal-change glomerulonephritis, which accounts for 75% of childhood nephrotic syndrome. If renal function deteriorates, treatment with cyclophosphamide and chlorambucil may be undertaken. IgM may be found in the mesangium in nephrotic syndrome as the mesangium acts as a 'scavenger' for filtered proteins but basement membrane deposition of IgM is not a characteristic feature of membranous glomerulonephritis.

4.24   A: Glomerular crescents may occur during episodes of macroscopic haematuria

In Europe, North America and Australia, IgA nephropathy is the most common form of glomerulonephritis. Only 15–20% of patients will eventually require dialysis. In common with all parenchymal renal disease, heavy proteinuria, eg more than 1 g/day, implies a worse prognosis. Other poor prognostic factors include abnormal renal function at presentation and frequent episodes of macroscopic haematuria. Episodes of macroscopic haematuria often occur in conjunction with infection and are characterised histologically by glomerular crescents. Loin pain occurs at such times due to renal parenchymal swelling and not because of bleeding.

4.25   E: Renal amyloidosis

Any cause of nephrotic syndrome may be complicated by renal vein thrombosis, especially membranous glomerulonephritis. Causes of hyperviscosity, including severe dehydration and myeloma, may also be complicated by renal vein thrombosis. There are clotting derangements that occur in amyloidosis which predispose to renal vein thrombosis. Renal carcinoma may invade the renal veins, which predisposes to thrombosis that may propagate into the inferior vena cava. Another risk factor for renal vein thrombosis is trauma to the vein, in particular cannulation.

4.26 B: Cystinosis

Noonan's syndrome is a hereditary form of hypertrophic cardiomyopathy; it is inherited in an autosomal dominant fashion and is not associated with any renal features. Von Hippel–Lindau syndrome is also inherited in an autosomal dominant fashion and manifests as spinal and cerebellar haemangiomas, renal carcinomas and retinal angiomas. Childhood polycystic kidney disease has autosomal recessive inheritance; the gene is localised to chromosome 6 and end-stage renal failure develops early in childhood – prognosis is poor. Vesico-ureteric reflux has a familial predisposition and in some families is inherited as an autosomal dominant trait. Cystinosis is inherited in an autosomal recessive fashion; cardinal features are short stature, chronic renal failure, eye and cardiac disease; Fanconi's syndrome occurring with proximal renal tubular acidosis may be caused by cystinosis.

4.27 A: History of childhood enuresis

Vesico-ureteric reflux often remains undiagnosed until presentation with chronic renal failure in adulthood. A history of bedwetting or repeated ill-defined childhood illnesses (urinary tract infections (UTIs)) may provide a clue. Evidence of UTI only occurs in approximately 40% of cases. Definitive investigation is a micturating cystourethrogram demonstrating reflux. Other useful investigations are intravenous urogram and radionuclide scanning; the kidneys are usually small and irregularly scarred. In some families there may be autosomal dominant inheritance of reflux disease. Once renal failure has occurred antireflux surgery is of limited benefit, except for symptomatic relief; antibiotics are indicated for urinary tract infections. Antineutrophil cytoplasmic antibody (ANCA) antibodies are not associated with vesico-ureteric reflux. It is important to investigate whether ANCA antibodies are raised against myeloperoxidase or PR3, which are associated with renal disease, or are raised against other neutrophil antigens such as lactoferrin.

4.28 C: Normal chest X-ray

Constitutional symptoms such as fever and night sweats occur in less than 20% of patients with urinary tuberculosis (TB). Sterile pyuria and/or microscopic haematuria only occur in approximately 25% of cases. Tuberculous cystitis causes frequency, urgency and dysuria; occasionally, urge incontinence necessitates urinary diversion or a bladder augmentation operation. There are no radiological signs of pulmonary tuberculosis (TB) in approximately 60% of cases. Raised serum angiotensin-converting enzyme (ACE) levels are a non-specific finding more commonly associated with sarcoidosis but serum angiotensin-converting enzyme (ACE) is also raised in lymphoma, pulmonary TB, asbestosis and silicosis.

4.29   D: Omeprazole

Of these drugs, omeprazole is the safest to use in renal failure, as its clearance is not affected by decreasing renal function. However, in patients who have received a renal transplant and are taking ciclosporin care is needed as omeprazole often leads to an increase in ciclosporin levels. Oxytetracycline exacerbates uraemia by increasing urea generation; all tetracyclines except doxycycline have this effect. Mesalazine can provoke interstitial nephritis through its sulphonamide component. Both ibuprofen and lisinopril may compromise renal perfusion in circumstances of volume depletion such as hypotension due to cardiac failure or in elderly patients with an intercurrent illness. Angiotensin-converting enzyme (ACE) inhibitors and angiotensin-II receptor antagonists must be used with caution in uraemia; they do have an antiproteinuria effect, which may slow the decline in renal function in addition to their hypotensive effect.

4.30   E: It is often associated with eosinophilia

Cholesterol emboli to the kidneys usually arise from an atheromatous aorta, and may be triggered by instrumentation (eg arteriography). They are found at autopsy in 17% of patients over 60 years of age, although they may be subclinical. The crystals usually lodge in arteries of diameter 150–300 mm, so complete renal infarction resulting in loin pain and haematuria is rare. There is typically evidence of microinfarcts elsewhere on the lower extremities, such as livedo reticularis and gangrenous toes. Leucocytosis, eosinophilia and reduced C3 are typical but not invariable findings.

4.31   B: Pulsed methylprednisolone may be used in treatment

Hepatitis C causes an immune complex-mediated membranoproliferative glomerulonephritis. The immunoglobulins are not cold agglutinins (antibodies causing agglutination of erythrocytes in the cold peripheries of the body), but cryoglobulins (types II and III mixed). Cryoglobulins are immunoglobulins that reversibly precipitate in the cold. One-third of patients exhibit spontaneous renal remission. Interferon-α is used in treatment; pulsed methylprednisolone and plasma exchange are also of value.

4.32 E: Mesangial widening, basement membrane thickening and capillary obliteration

Hyaline thrombi are found in monoclonal immunoglobulin deposition diseases, systemic lupus erythematosus (SLE) and thrombotic microangiopathies. The typical changes of membranous glomerulonephritis include capillary thickening, and spike-and-chain appearance of the basement membrane. Mesangial hypercellularity is seen in the proliferative glomerulopathies: poststreptococcal, mesangiocapillary, IgA/Henoch–Schönlein purpura, SLE, vasculitides, endocarditis. Green birefringence on staining with Congo red is a feature of amyloidosis.

4.33 E: Normal parathyroid hormone levels

The 1,25-dihydroxycholecalciferol is low or normal, not (as would be expected for the degree of hypophosphataemia) elevated. There is renal phosphate wasting, but glycosuria and aminoaciduria are absent. The condition is X-linked, but women may be affected by lyonisation.

4.34 B: Gastric ulceration is partly attributable to increased rate of *H. pylori* carriage

Cardiovascular death is the most important cause of death following transplantation. The risk of malignancy is much increased after transplantation; in more rare tumours the risk may be increased by a factor of 1000. Another predisposing risk factor for gastric ulceration is prednisolone therapy. With regard to infective complications, reverse barrier nursing is now considered unnecessary. A CMV-negative recipient should not receive a kidney from a CMV-positive donor, due to the risk of overwhelming infection (70–80% infection rate; 2% mortality in patients with disseminated disease). However, a CMV-positive recipient could receive a CMV-negative kidney. *Pneumocystis* infection typically occurs at 2–4 months.

4.35 C: Fluid intake should be 2–3 litres per day

Patients with severe renal impairment usually require fluid restriction to avoid peripheral oedema, pulmonary oedema and hypertension. However, in moderate renal impairment, it is usually important to drink 2–3 litres per day, to excrete the obligatory osmolar load (there is impairment of urinary concentration). There is evidence that moderate protein restriction may help slow progression of chronic renal failure, but severe protein restriction is likely to result in malnutrition and is mainly used to attenuate the symptoms of uraemia in patients unsuitable for dialysis. Patients with chronic renal failure are at increased risk of vascular disease; cholesterol intake needs to be controlled carefully. Patients on a phosphate-restriction diet need to limit their intake of dairy products.

4.36   C: HIV-associated nephropathy typically presents with nephrotic-range proteinuria

Renal involvement is rare (3% of autopsies of AIDS patients). The typical histological feature of HIV-associated nephropathy is focal or global capillary collapse. It may respond to zidovudine. The natural history is rapid progression to end-stage renal failure. Other features of HIV infection include hyponatraemia, hyperkalaemia and hypocalcaemia.

4.37   D: Penicillamine

Penicillamine works by converting cystine to cysteine-penicillamine, which is 50 times more soluble, hence reducing crystallisation. It should be used in conjunction with a high fluid intake. Alkalisation of the urine is theoretically beneficial, but does not appear to be clinically useful. Cysteamine may be used in the treatment of cystinosis.

4.38   B: Colestyramine

Colestyramine reduces urinary oxalate excretion in the case of enteric hyperoxaluria.

Spironolactone has no role in renal stone disease but thiazides may be used for their hypocalciuric effect.

4.39   E: Dipstick urinalysis and microscopy

The patient has rhabdomyolysis following the muscle damage caused by his prolonged convulsion. The low calcium, and markedly elevated potassium, creatinine and phosphate are highly suggestive of this diagnosis. Dipstick urinalysis will test positive for blood (due to the myoglobinuria), but urine microscopy will not demonstrate haematuria. Renal biopsy would confirm the diagnosis more definitively.

4.40   B: Antiglomerular basement membrane disease

The other causes of reduced CH50 in glomerulonephritis are shunt nephritis, type I mesangiocapillary glomerulonephritis, and infective endocarditis.

4.41 A: Adenoma sebaceum in a patient with microscopic haematuria

Accelerated or malignant hypertension, indicated funduscopically by grade 3 or 4 changes, may be an aetiological factor in renal failure, but hypertension is of course also an important consequence of renal failure. Adenoma sebaceum (facial angiofibromas) is a typical finding in tuberose sclerosis, a condition characterised by bilateral renal angiomyolipomas and cysts. Although hyperlipidaemia is seen in nephrotic syndrome, it is unlikely to have existed for long enough to cause arcus. Furthermore, it will not provide any aetiological clues, as it is a non-specific consequence of all causes of nephrotic syndrome. Cushing's syndrome is not typically associated with any renal disease. Up to 90% of patients with partial lipodystrophy develop progressive glomerulonephritis, most usually mesangiocapillary glomerulonephritis type II. A serum creatinine of 150 μmol/l with normal urinary sediment is an unlikely presentation of this condition.

4.42 A: Infection 2 weeks ago with α-haemolytic *Streptococcus*

Poststreptococcal glomerulonephritis is associated with group A α-haemolytic *Streptococcus*. The condition typically occurs 10 to 14 days after upper respiratory tract infection, or 3 weeks after a skin infection. It typically affects children aged 3 to 8 years old, boys more than girls. One-quarter of patients have normal renal function at presentation and 10% have no elevation of ASOT. The proteinuria is typically less than 2 g in 24 hours.

4.43 A: Eclampsia can occur without previous hypertension

Korotkoff phase V may not occur in pregnancy, so it is important to use phase IV. Blood pressure falls in the first trimester, reaches a nadir in the mid-trimester, and by term is comparable to non-pregnant blood pressure. This physiological fall is due to reduced vascular resistance, both by vasodilatation, and later due to the uteroplacental circulation. Cardiac output increases by about 40%. The accepted threshold for physiological proteinuria is 0.3 g/24 h. The risk of pre-eclampsia is 15 times greater for the first pregnancy than the second. Eclampsia occurs without any recognised pre-eclampsia in around 20% of cases.

4.44 A: Urinary protein excretion of 3 g/l, in conjunction with microscopic haematuria, may be attributable to strenuous exercise

Pathological levels of proteinuria are a reflection of: (a) glomerular pathology; (b) elevated plasma protein levels (overflow proteinuria); or (c) tubular damage (eg Fanconi's syndrome). Orthostatic proteinuria disappears during recumbency. Microalbuminuria is defined as proteinuria greater than the upper limit of normal (150 mg/24 h) but less than 100 mg/l (threshold for dipstick positivity). In young adults, the main causes of nephrosis are minimal-change disease, focal segmental glomerulosclerosis, proliferative glomerulonephritides, and Henoch–Schönlein disease. Membranous glomerulonephritis is more commonly seen in older patients, due to its association with malignancy.

4.45   C: A 60-year-old man who developed type 1 DM 43 years ago

Type 1 diabetes mellitus (DM): after development of diabetes, there is a lag period of about five years when development of nephropathy is rare. Thereafter, the annual incidence of the complication increases to a peak of 3% per year 15–17 years after development of diabetes. Patients who have had the disease for more than 35 years have a low risk of developing nephropathy. Type 2 DM: unlike type 1, the incidence of nephropathy rises steadily with time. The patient described in option D is likely to have had undetected diabetes for some time: such patients may present with, or rapidly develop, retinopathy and nephropathy. There is considerable racial heterogeneity with regard to incidence of nephropathy. Japanese and Pima Indians have a cumulative incidence of 50% after 20 years of diabetes, compared with 25% for Whites.

4.46   D: Water intake of 10 litres in 1 day would not result in hyponatraemia

Massive fluid volumes can be tolerated acutely in the normal patient. The hyponatraemia seen in psychogenic polydipsia is probably related to impairment of free water excretion. The obligated urine volume is approximately 0.8 l/day. It is important to be able to estimate the insensible losses of a patient accurately. In a normothermic patient, they will be approximately 0.5 l/day. However, this will rise significantly if the patient is pyrexial. The minimum required water intake is approximately 1.35 l/day. Water loss in stools is less than 0.05 l/day.

4.47   A: Cardiac/vascular

Anyone who answered B or E must have little faith in the nephrological service in this country! Malignancy is an important complication of transplantation. Infection is the second greatest cause of death, reflecting both the increased susceptibility of these patients to infection, and the instrumentation they require. However, vascular (including cardiac) causes of death account for 40–50% of all deaths in patients on dialysis. This is partly due to some of the conditions that result in ESRF (diabetes, renal artery disease) and to the increased number of elderly patients now receiving dialysis. However, renal failure itself increases the incidence of atherosclerotic disease, due to hypertension, lipid abnormalities, anaemia, and altered vessel wall characteristics.

4.48   A: A high proportion of distorted red cells suggests a glomerular origin

A family history of microscopic haematuria may provide a clue to Alport's syndrome or benign familial haematuria. Only major haematuria (> 50 ml/ 24 h) allows enough protein loss into the urine to give a positive result on dipstick testing. Presence of significant proteinuria should point the clinician firmly towards a renal origin. Haematuria is visible at a concentration of approximately 5 ml blood per litre of urine. Haematuria rarely results from standard warfarinisation in the absence of structural lesions.

4.49   C: Continuous veno-venous haemofiltration

To confirm a diagnosis of hepatorenal syndrome over prerenal azotaemia, it is often necessary to ensure that there is no reversibility in response to a fluid challenge, and/or to measure the central venous pressure as an estimate of vascular filling. However, once the diagnosis has been made, fluid and sodium restriction are crucial. Whereas orthotopic liver transplantation may be life saving, the kidneys are normal, and do not require transplantation. Although the renin–angiotensin system is implicated in the pathogenesis of hepatorenal syndrome, trials of the use of angiotensin-converting enzyme (ACE) inhibitors have resulted in severe hypotension. Some form of dialysis is often necessary to prevent life-threatening fluid overload, and to permit fluid administration of bicarbonate or hyperalimentation regimes. However, patients often exhibit too much cardiovascular instability to tolerate haemodialysis, and continuous veno-venous haemofiltration may be used instead.

4.50   B: Liver ultrasonography of patient

Neonatally, the two conditions are clinically indistinguishable. They are also indistinguishable on renal ultrasonography. Renal ultrasound on the parents will only be conclusive, in the case of a negative examination, if the parents are over the age of 30. There is no indication for IVP or renal biopsy. However, hepatic ultrasound should demonstrate biliary dysgenesis in the case of the recessive condition. Ultimately, genetic studies are most likely to be definitive.

REVISION CHECKLISTS

CLINICAL PHARMACOLOGY: REVISION CHECKLIST

Interactions/dose adjustment

- ☐ Drug interactions
- ☐ Pregnancy/breast-feeding
- ☐ Adverse effects – general
- ☐ Dose adjustment in renal failure
- ☐ Drugs in porphyria
- ☐ Polymorphism of drug metabolism
- ☐ Overdose/poisoning

Specific side-effects of drugs

- ☐ Asthma exacerbation
- ☐ Drugs causing hypothyroidism
- ☐ Gynaecomastia/ hyperprolactinaemia
- ☐ Hepatic enzyme inducers
- ☐ Hypokalaemia
- ☐ Aggravation of skin disorders
- ☐ Convulsions
- ☐ Haemolytic anaemia

Fundamental pharmacology

- ☐ Mechanisms of drug/antibiotic action
- ☐ Drug metabolism

Most frequently considered individual agents

- ☐ Antipsychotics/depressants
- ☐ ACE inhibitors
- ☐ Amiodarone
- ☐ Thiazides
- ☐ Anticonvulsants
- ☐ Digoxin
- ☐ Lithium
- ☐ Sulfasalazine
- ☐ Metronidazole
- ☐ Radio-iodine

Other 'topical' agents

- ☐ Azidothymidine (AZT)
- ☐ Antihypertensives
- ☐ Cimetidine
- ☐ Gentamicin
- ☐ Griseofulvin
- ☐ HMG Co-A reductase inhibitor
- ☐ Immunosuppressants
- ☐ L-dopa
- ☐ Metronidazole
- ☐ Nitrates
- ☐ NSAIDs
- ☐ Penicillamine
- ☐ Retinoic acid
- ☐ Warfarin
- ☐ Acetylcholinesterase inhibitors
- ☐ Antiretroviral therapy
- ☐ Magnesium (Asthma, eclampsia)

ENDOCRINOLOGY REVISION CHECKLIST

Diabetes and glycaemic control

- ☐ Diabetes
- ☐ Hypoglycaemia
- ☐ Glycosylated haemoglobin
- ☐ Hepatic gluconeogenesis
- ☐ Insulinoma

Adrenal disease

- ☐ Cushing's syndrome
- ☐ Addison's disease
- ☐ Congenital adrenal hyperplasia
- ☐ ACTH action
- ☐ Conn's disease

Thyroid disease

- ☐ Thyroxine action/metabolism/TFTs
- ☐ Thyroid cancer/nodule
- ☐ Graves' disease/exophthalmos
- ☐ Hypothyroidism

Parathyroid disease/calcium

- ☐ PTH/hyperparathyroidism

- ☐ Calcitonin
- ☐ Pituitary disease

Acromegaly

- ☐ Chromophobe adenoma
- ☐ Hyperprolactinaemia
- ☐ Hypopituitarism
- ☐ Pituitary hormones

Miscellaneous

- ☐ Polycystic ovarian syndrome/ infertility
- ☐ SIADH
- ☐ Short stature
- ☐ Weight gain/Prader–Willi syndrome
- ☐ Endocrine changes in anorexia
- ☐ Hirsutism
- ☐ Hormone physiology (including pregnancy)
- ☐ Sweating

GASTROENTEROLOGY: REVISION CHECKLIST

Liver disease

- ☐ Chronic liver disease
- ☐ Jaundice
- ☐ Primary biliary cirrhosis
- ☐ Gilbert's syndrome

- ☐ Hepatic mass/subphrenic abscess
- ☐ Alcohol and the liver
- ☐ Portal vein thrombosis

Small bowel disease/malabsorption

- ☐ Coeliac disease
- ☐ Malabsorption/protein-losing enteropathy
- ☐ Cholera toxin/gastroenteritis
- ☐ Carcinoid syndrome
- ☐ Whipple's disease
  (see also 'Crohn's disease' below)

Large bowel disorders

- ☐ Crohn's disease
- ☐ Ulcerative colitis/colonic carcinoma
- ☐ Irritable bowel syndrome
- ☐ Diarrhoea
- ☐ Inflammatory bowel disease – general
- ☐ Pseudomembranous colitis

Oesophageal disease

- ☐ Gastro-oesophageal reflux/tests
- ☐ Achalasia
- ☐ Dysphagia/oesophageal tumour
- ☐ Oesophageal chest pain

Stomach and pancreas

- ☐ Acute pancreatitis
- ☐ Gastric acid secretion
- ☐ Persistent vomiting
- ☐ Stomach cancer

Miscellaneous

- ☐ GI tract bleeding
- ☐ Abdominal X-ray
- ☐ GI hormones
- ☐ Physiology of absorption
- ☐ Recurrent abdominal pain
- ☐ Gall bladder disease

NEPHROLOGY: REVISION CHECKLIST

Nephrotic syndrome/related glomerulonephritis

- ☐ Nephrotic syndrome
- ☐ Membranous glomerulonephritis
- ☐ Minimal-change disease
- ☐ Hypocomplementaemia and glomerulonephritis
- ☐ Renal vein thrombosis
- ☐ Acute glomerulonephritis
- ☐ SLE nephritis

Renal failure

- ☐ Acute renal failure
- ☐ Acute versus chronic
- ☐ Chronic renal failure
- ☐ Haemolytic uraemic syndrome
- ☐ Rhabdomyolysis
- ☐ Anaemia in renal failure
- ☐ Contrast nephropathy

Urinary abnormalities

☐ Macroscopic haematuria

☐ Discoloration of the urine

☐ Nocturia

☐ Polyuria

Basic renal physiology

☐ Normal renal physiology/function

☐ Water excretion/urinary concentration

☐ Serum creatinine

Miscellaneous

☐ Distal renal tubular acidosis

☐ Renal papillary necrosis

☐ Diabetic nephropathy

☐ Analgesic nephropathy

☐ Polycystic kidney disease

☐ Renal calculi

☐ Renal osteodystrophy

☐ Retroperitoneal fibrosis

☐ Steroid therapy in renal disease

INDEX

Locators refer to question number.

CLINICAL PHARMACOLOGY

Index

ENDOCRINOLOGY

GASTROENTEROLOGY

NEPHROLOGY